Normal Values in Vision Science

Michael P. Kelly

Normal Values in Vision Science

Springer

Michael P. Kelly
School of Medicine
Duke University
Durham, NC, USA

ISBN 978-3-032-18206-7 ISBN 978-3-032-18207-4 (eBook)
https://doi.org/10.1007/978-3-032-18207-4

This Springer imprint is published by the registered company Springer Nature Switzerland AG
The registered company address is: Gewerbestrasse 11, 6330 Cham, Switzerland

for Evelyn

my love, my light, my life

Introduction

Recent advancements in gene therapy, stem cell therapy, and optogenetics are showing promise for treating eye disease, revolutionizing ophthalmology. In addition, Oculomics, a new field of study using ocular biomarkers to inform systemic disease, is in its infancy and holds promise for noninvasive early detection of a growing number of diseases including cardiovascular, kidney, and neurodegenerative disorders such as multiple sclerosis and Alzheimer's disease. Knowledge of normal values in vision science and ophthalmology is essential to identifying disease, especially as artificial intelligence (AI) and precision medicine play an increasingly important role in the future of healthcare. AI algorithms used for detecting disease will differentiate normal from abnormal using images and measurement data, including retinal layer thicknesses and optic nerve head parameters. Comprehensive data sets containing both normal and disease examples will enhance algorithmic accuracy and the ability to identify ocular and systemic disease sooner. Disease-staging will follow, ensuring those with urgent ocular pathology are flagged for faster intervention. Utilizing current and future formulas, treatment dosages of anti-vascular endothelial growth factor intravitreal injections could, for example, be tailored to an individual's exact vitreous volume. This precision may help minimize intraocular pressure spikes post injection, particularly in smaller eyes, reducing the risk of both over- and under-dosing and may also improve safety in procedures involving gas or silicone oil. Thus, knowing what is normal across diverse populations is key to ensuring accurate diagnoses and predictions. This book is a collection of normal vision science values maintained in notebooks over a decades-long career in clinical and research ophthalmic imaging and ophthalmology. I found my constantly expanding list to be a valuable resource, especially when working with subspecialties where my interactions were less frequent. This is not an exhaustive treatise on the eye and its functions; many detailed and valuable resources on that topic are readily available. This, rather, is a collection of normal values: measurements, volumes, rates, densities, velocities, amplitudes, frequencies, etc., with purposely limited accompanying text. Normal values can vary among individuals due to many factors (age, race, sex, device used, segmentations applied, etc.) and often have a range; the most generally accepted and used in current practice are included here. Although intended for trainees, this collection should prove useful to anyone in the vision science and ophthalmology fields. This information is of course subject to change as technology and global research speeds on, especially in the field of vision science and ophthalmology, underscoring the need for the reader to always confirm accuracy with additional sources prior to use to ensure the most currently accepted data will be applied. It is important to note that ophthalmic device manufacturers may use different acquisition methods leading to variations in the numeric values their devices report as compared to competitor devices. The information provided here should not be used to adjust device settings or guide research or treatment decisions. Due to reliance on ever-improving methods of ocular imaging to refine existing normative data, a section on Emerging Ocular Imaging Technology in vision science and ophthalmology is included.

Acknowledgments

Thank you to Kourtney Houser, MD, Associate Professor of Ophthalmology and Director of the Cornea Fellowship Program at Duke University Eye Center for reviewing the manuscript with such expertise.

Thank you to these generous individuals who expertly reviewed sections of the manuscript:

Oleg Alekseev, MD, PhD, Assistant Professor of Ophthalmology, Inherited Retinal Degenerations and Medical Retina, at Duke University Eye Center

Sophie Cai, MD, Assistant Professor of Ophthalmology, Surgical Retina The Wilmer Eye Institute, Johns Hopkins University

Kelly Donovan, MD, PhD, Duke University Eye Center

Madison Dunning, OD, Assistant Professor of Ophthalmology, Low Vision Rehabilitation Duke University Eye Center

Al-Hafeez Dhalla, PhD, Assistant Research Professor, Department of Biomedical Engineering at Duke University

Tanya Glaser, MD, Assistant Professor of Ophthalmology, Pediatric Ophthalmology and Strabismus, Duke University Eye Center

Michelle Go, MD, MSc, Assistant Professor of Ophthalmology, Pediatric Ophthalmology and Strabismus, Duke University Eye Center

Sidney Gospe, MD, Associate Professor of Ophthalmology, Neuro-Ophthalmology Duke University Eye Center

Divakar Gupta, MD, Associate Professor of Ophthalmology, Glaucoma Duke University Eye Center

Avital Lily Okrent Smolar, MD, Assistant Professor of Ophthalmology, Oculoplastics Duke University Eye Center

Ekaterina Semenova, MD, Assistant Professor of Ophthalmology, Ocular Oncology New York Eye and Ear of Mount Sinai, Icahn School of Medicine

Lejla Vajzovic, MD, Professor of Ophthalmology, Adult & Pediatric Vitreoretinal Diseases & Surgery, Duke University Eye Center

I am grateful to Scott Cousins, Cynthia Toth, Hilel Lewis, Everett Ai, and Howard Schatz for their invaluable mentorship. Their guidance, patience, friendship, and steadfast support have been foundational to my academic and professional journey.

Contents

About the Author

Michael P. Kelly served as Director of Duke University Eye Center's clinical and research imaging department from 2005 to 2023, and in a dual role as Director of Duke Eye Center Departmental Labs from 2012 to 2022, and now holds the position of Director of Duke Remote Diagnostic Screening. He previously directed the clinical and research imaging programs at West Coast Retina Medical Group, California Pacific Medical Center, Cleveland Clinic's Cole Eye Institute, and the Cincinnati Eye Institute. He stewarded these departments through the imaging and testing in dozens of national clinical trials, including the Anti-VEGF studies, the sustained-release and treat-and-extend trials, cytomegalovirus retinitis trials, the Collaborative Ocular Melanoma Study, and the Early Treatment of Diabetic Retinopathy Study. He is a Fellow and two-term Past President of the Ophthalmic Photographers' Society (OPS), has served on editorial boards for the American Academy of Ophthalmology (AAO) and the OPS, has published 48 peer-reviewed papers in 18 different ophthalmology and biomedical optics journals, served as guest editor for a special issue on imaging intraocular tumors, served as a subject matter expert for several ophthalmology journals, is a senior founding editor of the American Society of Retina Specialists retina image bank, and has written chapters in 4 textbooks. He has published works across four disciplines: ophthalmic imaging, biomedical optics, photography, and all subspecialties within ophthalmology. He has received the AAO Achievement Award and the AAO Secretariat Award. He has given more than two hundred lectures and has been an invited speaker twice at Bascom Palmer Eye Institute, twice at Ohio State University, and six times at the University of California at Berkeley, the University of California at San Francisco, Brown University, and the Cleveland Clinic. He has given talks for conferences at Harvard and Oxford, in Singapore, Chile, and the United Arab Emirates, and was the Keynote Speaker at Aalborg University's 2022 Oftalmologisk FotoSymposium in Denmark.

Chapter 1
Key Measurements of the Normal Adult Human Eye *At-a-Glance*

- Circumference of the eye: 75 mm
- Volume: 6.5–7.0 ml
- Weight of the eye: 7–8 gm
- Visual acuity: 20/20 in feet (6/6 in meters, 1.0 decimal in some countries)
- Visual field: 120° horizontally and 90–100° vertically
- Axial length: 22–25 millimeters (mm)
- Anterior chamber depth: 2.5 to 3 mm
- *Orbital* entrance: 35 mm wide × 40 mm high
- Orbital volume: 30 ml
- *Pupil* diameter: 2–4 mm in bright light, 4–8 mm in dim light
- Pupillary distance: 55–75 mm
- *Iris* diameter: horizontal 11.5–12 mm, vertical 10.5–12 mm
- Iris thickness: 0.5–0.6 mm
- Angle of the iris: 40–45° (between iris and cornea)
- *Corneal* diameter: 11.5 to 12 mm
- Corneal weight: 0.5 g
- Corneal curvature: 7.8 mm
- Corneal temperature: 32.0°–34.0 °C (89.6–93.2 F)
- Central corneal thickness: 520 to 550 microns
- Refractive index of the cornea: 1.376
- Refractive power of the cornea: +43D
- Refractive power of the corneal anterior surface: +48D
- Refractive power of the corneal posterior surface: −5D
- Corneal endothelial cell density: 2400–3000/mm squared
- Intraocular pressure range (IOP): 10–21 mmHg
- *Scleral* thickness, posterior: 1 mm
- Scleral thickness at equator: 0.6–0.8 mm
- Scleral thickness near the limbus: 0.8
- Scleral weight: 12 g

M. P. Kelly, *Normal Values in Vision Science*,
https://doi.org/10.1007/978-3-032-18207-4_1

- Scleral temperature: 35.0°–37.0 °C (95–98.6 °F)
- Scleral stiffness: 0.1–1.0 MPa
- Scleral radius of curvature: 7–10 mm
- Episcleral venous pressure (EVP): 6–9 mmHg
- *Conjunctival* sac volume: 35 μL
- Conjunctival temperature: 33.0°–34.0 °C (91.4–93.2 °F)
- *Ciliary body* width: 2–5 mm
- *Anterior chamber* central depth: 3–3.5 mm
- Anterior chamber aqueous humor volume: 250–300 μL
- Posterior chamber aqueous humor volume: 50–70 μL
- *Aqueous* humor weight: 0.25 g
- Aqueous humor volume: 0.30 mL
- Aqueous temperature: 36.0–37.0 °C (96.8–98.6 °F)
- Aqueous humor production: 2–2.5 μL/min
- Aqueous turnover rate: 1%/min
- *Lens* thickness: 4–5 mm [1]
- Lens weight: 135–255 mg
- Lens temperature: 36.0°–37.0 °C (96.8–98.6 °F)
- Lens refractive index: 1.39
- Lens refractive power: 16–17D
- *Vitreous* volume: 4 mL
- Vitreous weight: 15 g
- Vitreous temperature: 36.0°–37.0 °C (96.8–98.6 °F)
- *Retina* thickness at posterior pole: 0.56 mm
- Retina weight: 1.5 g
- Retina temperature: 36.5°–37.0 °C (97.7–98.6 °F)
- Diameter of *macula*: 5.5 mm and 15° of the visual field
- *Fovea* centralis diameter: 1.85 mm and 5 degrees of visual field
- Foveola diameter: 0.35 mm
- Light adaptation time: 5–10 min
- Number of *rods*: 120 million
- Density of rods in the periphery: 100,000–150,000 mm squared
- Density of rods in the central fovea: zero
- Dark adaptation times of rods: 30 min
- Accessory Inner Segment* (aIS): 120 million
- Number of *cones*: 6.5 million
- Density of cones in fovea (densest) location: 150,000–300,000/square mm
- Retinal Blood Flow Velocity: 3–4 cm/s in the central retinal artery
- Static Contrast Ratio: approximately 100:1, or 6.5 F-stops

*newly discovered structure supporting rods, 2025: https://doi.org/10.1038/s42003-025-07473-6

- Length of cones in the fovea: 25–40 microns
- Dark adaptation time of cones: 5 min
- *Choroidal* thickness at the fovea: 200–300 microns

- Choroidal thickness toward the ora serrata: 100–150 microns
- Choroidal weight: 2–3 g
- Choroidal temperature: 36.0°-37.0 °C (96.8–98.6 °F)
- Choroidal volume: 100–150 μL
- Choroidal vascular index (CVI): 65.61% ± 2.33%
- Suprachoroidal Space: 34.23 microns (at the fovea) [2]
- *Optic nerve* (ON) length: 47–50 mm [3]
- Intracranial ON length: 10 mm
- Intracanalicular length: 6–9 mm
- Intra-orbital ON length: 30 mm
- Intraocular ON length: 1 mm
- Optic disc diameter: 1.5 mm
- Number of nerve fibers: 1.2 million
- Optic chiasm size: 12 mm wide and 8 mm long
- Number of meibomian glands: 20–30 per lid
- Number of glands of Zeis: 2 per cilia
- Number of glands of Moll: 2–5 per eyelash follicle
- Number of glands of Krause in the fornices: 40–42 upper and 6–8 lower
- Number of glands of Wolfring in the tarsal border: 2–5 upper and 2–3 lower
- Length of lacrimal sac: 15 mm
- Rate of tear secretion: 1.2 ml/min
- pH of tear: 7.4
- Rate of blinking: 12–20 times per minute
- Tear Film Break-Up Time (tbut): >10 s
- Total dioptric power: +60D
- Nodal point: 7.2 mm behind the corneas anterior surface
- Principal point: 1-5 mm behind the corneas anterior surface
- Anterior focal point: 15.7 mm in front of the corneas anterior surface
- Posterior focal point: 24.4 mm behind the corneas anterior surface
- Saccadic Eye Movements: Normal Velocity: 200–700°/s [4–6]

These measurements provide a general overview and can vary among individuals.

Of Related Interest

In 2025, Duke University Eye Center researchers using enhanced imaging technology identified a previously unknown part of photoreceptor cells in the retina. Their finding challenges long-standing assumptions about the retina and opens new avenues for understanding vision and genetic eye diseases. https://doi.org/10.1038/s42003-025-07473-6

References

1. American Academy of Ophthalmology. Basic and clinical science course (BCSC). Section 3: clinical optics and vision rehabilitation. San Francisco: American Academy of Ophthalmology; 2022–2023.
2. Chang S, Hong A, Sazhnyev Y, Choy K, Durbin-Johnson B, Ko R, Sarabu N, Farsiu S, Emami-Naeini P, Moshiri A, Moussa K, Yiu G. Demographic and ocular factors associated with suprachoroidal space thickness in healthy eyes. Ophthalmol Sci. 2025;6(2):101006.
3. Riordan-Eva P. Fundamentals and principles of ophthalmology: basic and clinical science course companion. San Francisco: American Academy of Ophthalmology; 2022–2023. Chapter 2, Table 2-1. p. 49.
4. Miller D, Newman NJ, Biousse V, Kerrison JB, editors. Albert and Jakobiec's principles and practice of ophthalmology. 3rd ed. Philadelphia: Elsevier Saunders; 2008.
5. Yanoff M, Duker JS, editors. Ophthalmology. 5th ed. Philadelphia: Elsevier; 2018.
6. Tasman W, Jaeger EA, eds. Duane's ophthalmology. Philadelphia: Lippincott Williams & Wilkins; 2006. Chapter 4, Cornea and sclera, p. 85–102. Available from: https://www.duanesophthalmology.com

Chapter 2
Differences Between Normal Human Adult and Normal Infant Eye

The differences between the normal human adult eye and the normal infant eye extend far beyond mere size, encompassing structural, functional, and developmental distinctions. While the adult eye is fully mature in terms of anatomical proportions and visual capability, the infant eye is still undergoing critical postnatal development. Key variations include differences in axial length, corneal curvature, lens transparency and elasticity, retinal thickness, and the degree of myelination in the optic nerve. These factors influence visual acuity, refraction, and the eye's responsiveness to visual stimuli. Understanding the differences is crucial for diagnosing and managing ocular health at different stages of development.

Eye Size and Shape

- Axial Length:
- Infant: Typically, shorter, around 16–17 millimeters (mm) at birth [1].
- Adult: Generally, longer, around 22–24 mm. The eye length increases during childhood as part of normal development.
- Corneal Diameter:
- Infant: Approximately 9–10 mm
- Adult: Around 11–12 mm [2]
- Pupillary distance (PD):
- Adult: 55–75 mm
- Infant: 40–50 mm

M. P. Kelly, *Normal Values in Vision Science*,
https://doi.org/10.1007/978-3-032-18207-4_2

Corneal Measurements

- Central Corneal Thickness (CCT):
- Infant: CCT in 6 to 23 months, 538 +/− 40 microns; 2–4 years, 546 +/− 41 μm; 5–9 years, 566 +/− 48 μm; and 10–18 years, 554 +/− 35 μm [3].
- Adult: Typically, 500–550 μm. Thickness can vary slightly with age and eye condition.
- Corneal Curvature:
- Infant: Generally steeper, with a higher average curvature.
- Adult: Typically, less steep due to growth and changes in the corneal shape over time.

Lens

- Lens Power:
- Infant: Higher, due to a more rounded and thicker lens. The power of the lens decreases with age.
- Adult: Lower power due to changes in lens curvature and thickness.
- Lens Thickness:
- Infant: Thicker lens, contributing to higher refractive power.
- Adult: Thinner lens with reduced refractive power due to natural aging.

Visual Acuity

- Infant:
- At Birth: VA is around 20/400 or worse.
- By Age 5–7: VA improves to approximately 20/25 to 20/40, approaching adult levels.
- Adult Normal VA: 20/20 [4]

Ocular Motility

- Saccadic Movements:
- Infant: Peak velocities in infants can be lower compared to adults.
- Adult: Faster and more accurate saccades, with peak velocities around 300–700° per second (°/s).
- Smooth Pursuit:

- Infant: Limited smooth pursuit abilities. Pursuit speeds are generally slower, around 15–30° per second (°/s).
- Adult: More effective pursuit with speeds up to 30–60° per second (°/s) [5]

Pupillary Responses

- Pupillary Light Reflex:
- Infant: The reflex is present but can be less pronounced. Latency is typically longer compared to adults.
- Adult: More rapid and pronounced pupillary light reflex.

Pupil Size:

- Infant: Generally smaller, around 2–4 mm in diameter.
- Adult: Typically, 2–8 mm, varying with light conditions and age [6].

Retinal Structure and Function

- Retinal Thickness:
- Infant: The retinal layers are thinner at birth and develop over time.
- Adult: Thicker retinal layers, with normal values around 250–300 microns (μm) depending on the specific retinal layer.
- Visual Development:
- Infant: Visual acuity and retinal processing capabilities are still developing. Full maturation of visual pathways occurs about age 7 years.
- Adult: Fully developed visual pathways with mature visual processing capabilities.

Tear Production

- Infant:
- Tear Production: Lower tear production in infants, which increases as they grow.
- Tear Film Stability: Tear film break-up time (TBUT) may be shorter in infants.
- Adult:
- Tear Production: Higher and more stable tear production with a more consistent TBUT.

Postnatal Development of Eye Structures

Retina and Fovea

- Foveal Maturation: At birth, the fovea is underdeveloped. Cone photoreceptors in this region continue to elongate and become more densely packed over the first 4–5 years, enhancing visual acuity. Full maturation may extend up to 7–10 years of age.
- Retinal Layers: The layering and synaptic connections within the retina continue to refine postnatally, contributing to improved visual processing.

Optic Nerve and Visual Pathways

- Myelination: The optic nerve and visual pathways undergo significant myelination after birth, which is crucial for efficient signal transmission. This process continues for several months postnatally.

Lens

- Growth: The lens continues to grow throughout life by adding new lens fibers. Rapid growth occurs during early childhood, contributing to changes in refractive properties.

Cornea

- Curvature and Thickness: The cornea undergoes changes in curvature and thickness after birth, reaching adult dimensions typically by 1–2 years of age.

Iris and Pupil

- Pigmentation: Iris pigmentation increases during the first year of life, often leading to changes in eye color.
- Pupil Function: The neural control of pupil responses matures postnatally, improving light reflexes.

Sclera and Orbit

- Scleral Development: The sclera thickens and becomes more opaque after birth.
- Orbital Growth: The bony orbit expands significantly during the first 2 years, accommodating the growing eye.

Lacrimal System

1. Tear Production: While the lacrimal glands are present at birth, functional tear production typically begins between 2 weeks and 3 months of age. [7, 8]

Further Reading

Edward DP, Kaufman LM. Anatomy, development, and physiology of the visual system. Pediatr Clin N Am. 2003;50(1):1–23.

Eustis HS, Guthrie ME. Postnatal development. In: Pediatric ophthalmology and strabismus. Springer; 2007.

Van Cruchten S, et al. Pre- and postnatal development of the eye: a species comparison. Birth Defects Res C Embryo Today. 2017;109(19):1540–67.

References

1. Groot ALW, Lissenberg-Witte BI, van Rijn LJ, Hartong DT. Meta-analysis of ocular axial length in newborns and infants up to 3 years of age. Surv Ophthalmol. 2022;67(2):342–52. https://doi.org/10.1016/j.survophthal.2021.05.010. Epub 2021 Jun 9
2. Tucker SM, Enzenauer RW, Levin AV, et al. Corneal diameter, axial length, and intraocular pressure in premature infants. Ophthalmology. 1992;99(8):1296–300.
3. Hussein MA, Paysse EA, Bell NP, Coats DK, Wallace DK, Steele EA, et al. Corneal thickness in children. Am J Ophthalmol. 2004;138(5):744–8. https://doi.org/10.1016/j.ajo.2004.05.070.
4. Birch EE, Birch DG, Hoffman DR, Hale L. Postnatal development of visual acuity. Vis Neurosci. 1993;10(2):289–97.
5. Leigh RJ, Zee DS. The neurology of eye movements. 5th ed. Oxford: Oxford University Press; 2015. p. 193–5.
6. Brodsky MC. Pediatric neuro-ophthalmology. 2nd ed. New York: Springer; 2010. p. 78.
7. Ingraham HJ. Basic and clinical science course. Section 1: update on general medicine. San Francisco: American Academy of Ophthalmology; 2022–2023.
8. Brar VS. Basic and clinical science course. Section 2: fundamentals and principles of ophthalmology. San Francisco: American Academy of Ophthalmology; 2022–2023.

Chapter 3
Genetic and Ethnic Factors

Genetic and ethnic factors play a significant role in determining the normal structure and function of the eye. These differences affect various eye measurements and increase or decrease the risk for certain vision conditions. Genetic factors play a crucial role in the development of refractive errors. East Asians have a higher genetic predisposition to myopia and genetic variants have been identified that are linked to refractive errors, including mutations in genes associated with eye growth and the development of myopia. Genetic variants related to AMD are more common in Caucasians, and glaucoma-related genetic variants are more prevalent in African populations. Understanding these variations helps in diagnosing and managing eye diseases more accurately across different populations [1].

Refractive Errors and Ethnicity

Different ethnic groups show distinct patterns in refractive errors such as myopia, hyperopia, and astigmatism:

- Myopia
  - East Asians: Most affected; high myopia is especially common due to genetic predisposition.
  - Caucasians: Common but usually develops in adulthood and is less severe.
  - Africans: Lower prevalence than East Asians and Caucasians.
  - South Asians (e.g., India): Relatively common.
- Hyperopia
  - More common in Caucasians than in East Asian or African populations.
- Astigmatism

M. P. Kelly, *Normal Values in Vision Science*,
https://doi.org/10.1007/978-3-032-18207-4_3

- Caucasians: Moderate prevalence, usually regular astigmatism.
- East Asians: Common, but higher rates of irregular and severe cases.
- Africans: High prevalence of both regular and irregular forms [2].

Corneal Characteristics

- Corneal Thickness
  - Caucasians: ~540–550 microns
  - East Asians: Similar to Caucasians (~540 microns)
  - Africans: Slightly thinner (~530–540 microns)
- Corneal Curvature
  - Africans: Steeper
  - East Asians: Flatter
  - Caucasians: Intermediate

Intraocular Pressure (IOP)

- Africans: Typically have the highest IOP levels.
- East Asians: Lower than Africans but higher than Caucasians.
- Caucasians and South Asians: Tend to have similar, lower average IOP.

Axial Length

Axial length is closely linked to refractive errors (longer eyes = myopia; shorter = hyperopia).

- East Asians: Longest axial length, greater risk for myopia.
- Caucasians: Similar axial length to East Asians.
- Africans: Generally shorter axial length.
- South Asians: In between East Asians and Caucasians [3].

Optic Nerve Head and Retina

- Optic Nerve Head Size
  - Caucasians: Largest

    - Africans: Slightly smaller
    - East Asians: Smallest

- Retinal Nerve Fiber Layer (RNFL)

    - Thicker in Caucasians and Africans
    - Thinner in East Asians

- Macular Thickness

    - Caucasians: Thick
    - Africans: Also relatively thick
    - East Asians: Thin [4]

Pupil Size and Reaction

- East Asians: Generally smaller pupils.
- Caucasians: Larger pupils at baseline.
- Africans: Similar baseline size to Caucasians but show greater dilation in response to light.

Genetic Predispositions to Eye Conditions

- Myopia.

    - Most common in East Asians; linked to gene variants affecting eye growth.

- Age-Related Macular Degeneration (AMD).

    - Caucasians have a higher frequency of AMD-related mutations.

- Glaucoma.

    - Africans show a higher prevalence of glaucoma-associated genetic mutations.

Of Related Interest There is a lack of representation of most racial and ethnic populations in clinical trials in ophthalmology. In 2017, Roche/Genentech began to introduce a range of initiatives to improve the diversity of participants in phase 3 trials for ophthalmology.

Scott AW, Brown J, Prager AJ, et al. Racial and ethnic diversity in ophthalmology: a meta-analysis of industry-sponsored phase 3 clinical trials from a single company. Eye Open. 2025;1:3. https://doi.org/10.1038/s44440-025-00002-8.

References

1. Tham YC, Li X, Wong TY, Quigley HA, Aung T, Cheng CY. Global prevalence of glaucoma and projections of glaucoma burden through 2040: a systematic review and meta-analysis. Ophthalmology. 2014;121(11):2081–90. https://doi.org/10.1016/j.ophtha.2014.05.013. Epub 2014 Jun 26
2. Wojciechowski R. Nature and nurture: the complex genetics of myopia and refractive error. Clin Genet. 2011;79(4):301–20. https://doi.org/10.1111/j.1399-0004.2010.01592.x. Epub 2010 Dec 13
3. Amini N, Nowroozzadeh MH, Mirzajani A, et al. Corneal thickness profile and its association with ethnicity, refractive error, and ocular biometrics. J Cataract Refract Surg. 2010;36(2):287–91. https://doi.org/10.1016/j.jcrs.2009.08.042.
4. Bressler NM, Silva JC, Bressler SB, et al. Age-related macular degeneration in ethnic minorities: current status and future directions. Retina. 2003;23(4):S15–7. https://doi.org/10.1097/00006982-200308001-00004.

Chapter 4
The Ocular Cells

The human eye comprises a complex and highly specialized array of cells, each playing a critical role in maintaining vision and ocular health. From the transparent, protective epithelial cells of the cornea to the highly sensitive photoreceptors in the retina, ocular cells are uniquely adapted to support the eye's optical and neural functions. These cells contribute to processes such as light transmission, immune defense, nutrient transport, and signal transduction.

Cell Sizes and Locations

Cell type	Location	Size
Photoreceptors	Retina (outer layer)	
– Rods	Peripheral retina	~2 μm wide, ~40–60 μm long
– Cones	Fovea centralis	~1.5–4 μm wide, ~40–60 μm long
Retinal pigment epithelium (RPE)	Under photoreceptors	~10–14 μm across, polygonal shape [1]
Bipolar cells	Retina (middle layer)	~10–15 μm cell body
Horizontal cells	Retina	~10–15 μm cell body
Amacrine cells	Retina	~10–20 μm diameter
Ganglion cells	Retina (inner layer)	Varies: ~10–30 μm (cell body); some up to 50 μm [2]
- Ganglion cell axons	Form optic nerve	~0.8–1.2 μm in diameter (average)
Müller glia	Spans retina thickness	~2–10 μm wide, ~100–120 μm long
Corneal epithelial cells	Cornea (outer layer)	~25–50 μm in diameter [3]
Corneal endothelial cells	Cornea (inner layer)	~18–20 μm wide, ~5 μm thick [4]

M. P. Kelly, *Normal Values in Vision Science*,
https://doi.org/10.1007/978-3-032-18207-4_4

Cell type	Location	Size
Lens epithelial cells	Front surface of lens	~5–10 μm thick, varies in shape
Lens fiber cells	Inside lens	~10 μm wide, many mm long (spindle-shaped)
Conjunctival cells	Eye surface (mucosa)	~15–20 μm wide
Iris pigment cells	Iris	~10–20 μm wide
Limbal stem cells	Corneal edge (limbus)	~10–15 μm diameter

Minimum Critical Cell Densities and Aging

Endothelial Cells

Corneal endothelial cell density is considered to be between 1500 and 3500 cells per square millimeter (cells/mm^2), although this can vary with age; density is highest at birth with approximately 3000 cells/mm^2 and tends to decrease to 2500 cells/mm^2 in adulthood.

- Normal Range:

  1500 to 3500 cells/mm^2.

- Age-Related Changes:

  Density decreases with age, starting from approximately 3000 cells/mm^2 at birth to about 2500 cells/mm^2 in adulthood.

- Minimum Critical Density:

  The minimum critical density to maintain the pumping function of the endothelium is 400–500 cells/mm^2.

- Factors Influencing Density and/or Function:

  Systemic diseases, ocular diseases, and ophthalmic interventions [5].

Rods

- Normal Range:

  Approximately 92 to 120 million rod cells per retina. Rod density peaks at about 150,000 to 180,000 cells/mm^2 in a ring around the fovea. The fovea is absent of rods.

- Age-Related Changes:

Rod density gradually decreases with age, especially in the peripheral retina with a decline of 30–50% by the age of 80, primarily due to retinal pigment epithelium degeneration. Night vision (scotopic vision) worsens with age due to rod loss and slower dark adaptation.

- Minimum Critical Density:

For functional scotopic (low-light) vision, estimates suggest that with density below ~10,000–20,000 cells/mm^2, scotopic vision degrades.

- Factors Influencing Density and/or Function:

Genetics, conditions such as retinitis pigmentosa, age-related macular degeneration, or glaucoma, vitamin A deficiency can impair or damage rods, chronic exposure to bright light or cUV radiation may accelerate rod degeneration. Retinal detachment can reduce local rod density.

Cones

- Normal Range:

Approximately 6 to seven million cones per retina. The central fovea has the highest density with up to 150,000 to 300,000 cones/mm^2. Density is significantly less outside the fovea. Cones are present throughout the retina but less in the periphery.

- Age-Related Changes:

Cone density is stable in the fovea with aging. There is a modest decline beyond the fovea.
Function Declines: cone function may decline due to intrinsic degeneration such as in cone dystrophy, or secondary to neurovascular diseases as in diabetic retinopathy, ischemia, and degeneration of the retinal pigment epithelium.

- Minimum Critical Density:

Approximately 30,000–50,000 cones/mm^2 in the foveal region. Visual acuity, color vision, and fine detail perception begin to degrade below this threshold.

- Factors Influencing Density and/or Function:

Genetics, ocular diseases including glaucoma and macular degeneration, systemic disorders including diabetes and neurodegenerative conditions.

Retinal Ganglion Cells (RGCs)

Approximately 1.1 to 1.5 million RGCs per eye with the highest density in the parafoveal region, up to 30,000–40,000 cells/mm^2. Density decreases towards the periphery, with none in the foveal pit.

- Age-Related Changes:

  RGCs decrease with age, starting in early adulthood with a loss rate estimated at 0.3–0.6% per year with a 15–30% loss by the age of 80. Resulting in diminished visual field sensitivity and contrast sensitivity, especially in dim light.

- Minimum Critical Density:

  Approximately 6000–8000 RGCs/mm^2 in the central retina is needed for maintaining functional high-resolution vision. Visual acuity, visual field, and contrast sensitivity can diminish significantly when below this threshold.

- Factors Influencing Density and/or Function:

  Genetics, glaucoma, chronically high intraocular pressure, optic neuritis, hypertension, multiple sclerosis, or Alzheimer's disease [6, 7].

Bipolar Cells

- Normal Range:

  40 to 50 million bipolar cells per retina with highest densities near the parafoveal region.

- Age-Related Changes:

  Relatively resistant to aging. Bipolar cells may undergo metabolic stress or apoptosis in diabetes and diabetic retinopathy.

- Minimum Critical Density:

  Functional thresholds are at approximately 20,000–30,000 cells/mm^2 in central retina to maintain normal photopic and scotopic signal pathways.

- Factors Influencing Density and/or Function:

  Genetics, and inherited or acquired retinal diseases.

Horizontal Cells

- Normal Range:

1 to two million horizontal cells.

- Age-Related Changes:

  Relatively stable.

- Minimum Critical Density:

  There is not a specific minimum density established.

- Factors Influencing Density and/or Function:

  Genetics

Mueller Cells (A Type of Glial Cell Found in the Retina)

- Normal Range:

Estimated to be 5–seven million per retina.

Density: In the central retina, the density of Mueller cells can range between 3000 to 4000 cells per millimeter squared in the fovea, decreasing in peripheral regions. This density may vary slightly based on factors like age and retinal health.

- Age-Related Changes:

Thought to be relatively stable throughout life but can decrease with aging more so in the peripheral retina, and some diminished function of the cells with aging.

- Minimum Critical Density:

The minimum critical density of Mueller cells is not established.

- Factors Influencing Density and/or Function:

Genetic predispositions can affect both density and functions of the cells, inflammation secondary to uveitis, and medications including Tamoxifen and Hydroxychloroquine.

Lens Epithelial Cells

- Normal Range:
- one million cells cover the anterior surface of the lens.
- Density:
  - 4000–6000 cells/mm^2 in young adults.
- Age-Related Changes:
- LEC density decreases gradually with age.

  - Decreased ability to regulate homeostasis and protect against oxidative stress.
  - Contributes to lens opacification (cataracts) and stiffening (presbyopia).

- Minimum Critical Density:
- Studies suggest that below 2000–2500 cells/mm^2 in the central region, the ability to maintain lens transparency and repair is compromised.

  - Reduced density correlates with increased risk of age-related cataract formation.

- Factors Influencing Density:

UV light exposure, smoking, and poor antioxidant defense accelerate LEC loss, genetics, diabetes, trauma during cataract surgery could lead to LEC loss or abnormal proliferation resulting in posterior capsular opacification.

Lens Fiber Cells

Normal Range:

- The total number is estimated to be in the tens of millions; the exact count is not possible to define because lens fibers are continuously added throughout life.
- Age-Related Changes:

  - Lens fiber cells are continually produced but never shed. The lens grows in thickness and mass with age.
  - Central fibers become more compacted and less elastic, contributing to presbyopia and increased rigidity.
  - Accumulation of oxidatively damaged proteins leading to cataract formation.

- Minimum Critical Density:

  - There is no defined minimum density because fiber cells accumulate rather than decrease.

- Factors Influencing Density and/or Function.
- Chronic UV exposure, smoking, diabetes, genetics, nutrition deficiencies, and low antioxidant levels promote damage to crystallins [8, 9].

Cell Regeneration Rates

Human ocular cells vary in how quickly they regenerate/replace themselves. Most of the regenerative activity in the human eye is limited to surface and barrier cells, as in the corneal epithelium and conjunctiva, while deeper structures such as the lens and retinal cells are mostly incapable of regeneration.

Retinal Ganglion and Bipolar Cells: replacement rate: do not regenerate.

Cell Types That Replace Themselves or Possess Some Regenerative Capacity

Corneal Epithelium.
Rapid renewal: 7–10 days

- Limited repair via cell enlargement, not division. Endothelial cells do not divide but can migrate to cover damaged areas.

Corneal Endothelium

- Limited repair via cell enlargement.

Conjunctival Epithelium

- Replenished regularly.

Limbal Stem Cells

- Constantly supply new corneal epithelial cells.

Iris Pigment Epithelium

- Very limited regeneration, but not functional.

Cells with poor or absent mitotic (regenerative) potential.
Photoreceptors

- Outer segments renew daily, but cell bodies do not regenerate.

Retinal Ganglion Cells and Bipolar Cells

- Do not regenerate.

Retinal Pigment Epithelium (RPE)

- Low turnover.

Lens Fibers

- Central fibers last a lifetime; no turnover.

Müller Glia (Retina)

- Muller cells proliferate and can cause gliosis, occurring in disease.

Physical Limits of Detection in Human Eye Cells

Photon Detection Limit

- Rods are so sensitive they can respond to just 1 photon under ideal conditions, however due to neural noise it usually takes 5–7 photons for a person to consciously detect light.
- Cones require hundreds of photons to trigger a signal.

Wavelength Sensitivity

- Visible range: ~380–740 nm.
  - Blue cones (S-cones): ~420 nm.
  - Green cones (M-cones): ~530 nm.
  - Red cones (L-cones): ~560 nm.
- Outside this range:
  - UV (<380 nm): is mostly blocked by the lens and cornea, though children see slightly more UV than adults.
  - Infrared (>740 nm): cannot be seen as there is not sufficient energy to trigger photoreceptors.

Spatial Resolution (Detail)

- Best acuity: ~20/10 in rare individuals to 20/20.
- Foveal cones can distinguish features as small as 0.2 arcminutes (1/300 of a degree).
- Outside the fovea resolution drops rapidly.

Temporal Resolution (Flicker Fusion)

- The eye can detect flicker up to:
  - ~60 Hz and up to 75–90 Hz in some individuals, especially under bright light or in the peripheral retina.
- Rods respond slower than cones, affecting low-light flicker perception.

Contrast Sensitivity

- Human vision can detect contrast differences as low as 0.5% under ideal conditions.
- Retinal ganglion cells specialize in contrast detection via center-surround receptive fields.

Dynamic Range (Light Intensity)

- The human eye can operate across a range of ~10^{12}-fold difference in light intensity, from starlight to sunlight due to:
  - Pupil dilation.
  - Photoreceptor adaptation.
  - Neural processing.
- Only about 4–5 log units (10,000–100,000×) of brightness can be processed.

Motion Detection

- Highly sensitive to motion in the peripheral vision.
- Can detect movement as small as 1–2 arcminutes per second.
- Certain retinal ganglion cells (e.g., parasol cells) specialize in detecting rapid motion [10, 11].

Of Related Interest

In 2025, Biomedical engineers at Duke University developed an AI-powered imaging system, Deep compressed multichannel adaptive optics scanning light Ophthalmoscope (DCAOSLO), that visualizes individual retinal cells with unprecedented clarity and speed. This innovation could revolutionize early diagnosis and monitoring of neurological, cardiovascular, diabetic, and retinal diseases, as retinal cells act as surrogates for studying brain-related conditions.

Park J, et al. Deep compressed multichannel adaptive optics scanning light ophthalmoscope. Sci Adv. 2025; https://doi.org/10.1126/sciadv.adr5912.

References

1. Grünert U, Martin PR, Wissinger B. Cell types and cell circuits in the human retina. Prog Retin Eye Res. 2020;75:100800. https://doi.org/10.1016/j.preteyeres.2020.100800.

2. Kim US, Mahroo OA, Yu-Wai-Man C, Mollon JD. Retinal ganglion cells—diversity of cell types and clinical relevance. Front Neurol. 2021;12:661938. https://doi.org/10.3389/fneur.2021.661938.
3. Patel DV, McGhee CNJ, Wu F, Sherwin T, Craig JP, Coroneo MT. Comparison of human corneal cell density by age and corneal region using in vivo confocal microscopy. BMC Ophthalmol. 2016;16:129. https://doi.org/10.1186/s12886-016-0290-5.
4. Prydal JI, Ødegaard SA, Doughty MJ, Zaman ML, Hovding G. Normal human keratocyte density and corneal thickness measured by confocal microscopy in vivo. Eye (Lond). 1998;12(Pt 6):936–41. https://doi.org/10.1038/eye.1998.247.
5. Murphy C, Wilson RS. Effect of age on the endothelial cell count in the normal human cornea. Br J Ophthalmol. 1984;68(3):147–51. https://doi.org/10.1136/bjo.68.3.147.
6. Gao H, Hollyfield JG. Aging of the human retina: differential loss of neurons and retinal pigment epithelial cells. Invest Ophthalmol Vis Sci. 1992;33(1):1–17.
7. Curcio CA, Millican CL, Allen KA, Kalina RE. Photoreceptor topography in ageing and age-related maculopathy. Invest Ophthalmol Vis Sci. 1993;34(12):3278–96.
8. Zhu JH, Chen J, Zhang Y, et al. A single-cell transcriptomic atlas of human lens epithelium: cell subclasses, aging signatures, and maintenance of homeostasis. Stem Cell Res Ther. 2025;16:44. https://doi.org/10.1186/s13287-025-04436-w.
9. Vaghefi E, Donaldson PJ, Grey AC, et al. Age-associated changes in human lens fiber cell morphology. Aging Cell. 2020;19(1):e13025. https://doi.org/10.1111/acel.13025.
10. Fong SW, Chirila T, Ingraham HJ. Basic and clinical science course. Section 1: update on general medicine. San Francisco: American Academy of Ophthalmology; 2022–2023.
11. Brar VS. Basic and clinical science course. Section 2: fundamentals and principles of ophthalmology. San Francisco: American Academy of Ophthalmology; 2022–2023.

Chapter 5
Subjective Clinical Indices

Anterior Chamber (AC) Cells & Flare Grading (SUN Working Group Standard) in the evaluation of anterior uveitis [1].

AC Cells (per high-power field).

Grade	Description	Cells count
0	None	< 1
0.5+	Trace	1–5
1+	Mild	6–15
2+	Moderate	16–25
3+	Marked	26–50
4+	Severe	>50

AC Flare (Protein Content in Aqueous).

Grade	Description
0	None
1+	Faint (barely detectable)
2+	Moderate (iris/lens clear)
3+	Marked (iris/lens hazy)
4+	Intense (fibrin or plastic aqueous)

Corneal Staining (Oxford Scale) in the evaluation of exposure keratopathy, dry eye, contact lens fit [2].

Grade	Description
0	No staining
1	Minimal (1–5 dots)
2	Mild (6–15 dots)

M. P. Kelly, *Normal Values in Vision Science*,
https://doi.org/10.1007/978-3-032-18207-4_5

Grade	Description
3	Moderate (16–30 dots)
4	Marked (31–100 dots)
5	Severe (>100 dots, coalesced areas)

Cataract Grading (LOCS III—Lens Opacities Classification System III).

- Scale is continuous from 0.1 to 6.9, but commonly rounded to integers in clinical settings [3].

Grade	Range (LOCS III)
1	Minimal opacity
2	Mild
3	Moderate
4	Marked
5+	Severe

Optic Disc Cupping (Cup-to-Disc Ratio, CDR. Also for asymmetry of >0.2 between eyes). In the evaluation of glaucoma.

CDR	Description
≤0.3	Normal
0.4–0.6	Suspicious
≥0.7	Likely glaucomatous
≥0.9	Severe glaucomatous damage

Relative Afferent Pupillary Defect (RAPD) in the evaluation of optic nerve disorders, optic pathway disorders, and some retinal disorders such as vein and artery occlusions.

Grade	Description
+1	Weak initial constriction → dilation
+2	No initial constriction → dilation
+3	Immediate dilation
+4	Fixed dilated pupil, no response

Fluorescein Tear Break-Up Time (TBUT) in the evaluation of tear film [4].

TBUT	Interpretation
>10 sec	Normal
5–10 sec	Borderline
<5 sec	Abnormal (dry eye)

Vitreous Cells or Haze (SUN Vitreous Haze Scale).

Grade	Description
0	Clear
0.5+	Trace
1+	Slight haze

Grade	Description
2+	Moderate haze
3+	Marked haze, details obscured
4+	Optic nerve barely visible

Subjective Clinical Indices Summary Table

Parameter	Scale/grade	Range
AC cells	0 to 4+	<1 to >50 cells
AC flare	0 to 4+	None to fibrin/plastic
Corneal staining	0 to 5	No to severe (Oxford scale)
Cataracts (LOCS III)	1 to 6.9	Minimal to severe
Cup-to-Disc Ratio	0.1 to ≥0.9	Normal to advanced glaucoma
RAPD	+1 to +4	Weak response to fixed pupil
TBUT	<5 to >10 s	Dry eye to normal
Vitreous haze	0 to 4+	Clear to obscured disc [5, 6]

References

1. Jabs DA, Nussenblatt RB, Rosenbaum JT, SUN Working Group. Standardization of uveitis nomenclature for reporting clinical data: results of the first international workshop. Am J Ophthalmol. 2005;140(3):509–16. https://doi.org/10.1016/j.ajo.2005.03.057.
2. Bron AJ, Evans VE, Smith JA, Nuffield Laboratory of Ophthalmology, University of Oxford. Grading of corneal and conjunctival staining in the context of other dry eye tests. Cornea. 2003;22(7):640–50. https://doi.org/10.1097/00003226-200310000-00008.
3. Chylack LT Jr, Wolfe JK, Singer DM, Leske MC, Bullimore MA, Bailey IL, Friend J, McCarthy D, Wu SY, Longitudinal Study of Cataract Study Group. The lens opacities classification system III. Arch Ophthalmol. 1993;111(6):831–6. https://doi.org/10.1001/archopht.1993.01090060119035.
4. Norn MS. The tear break up time (TBUT) test: its origin and clinical significance. Optom Vis Sci. 1970;47(3):865–75.
5. Fong SW, Chirila T, Ingraham HJ. Basic and clinical science course. Section 1: update on general medicine. San Francisco: American Academy of Ophthalmology; 2022–2023.
6. Brar VS. Basic and clinical science course. Section 2: fundamentals and principles of ophthalmology. San Francisco: American Academy of Ophthalmology; 2022–2023.

Chapter 6
Additional Visual Experience Measures

Disability glare, discomfort glare, visual range, photo-stress recovery time, and chromatic contrast are all measures of visual performance that may be affected by light filtering.

Disability Glare is a reduction in visual performance due to light scattering, reducing contrast and resulting in difficulty visualizing objects, for example, with on-coming automobile headlights at night [1].

- Measured in terms of veiling luminance (Lv) in cd/m^2 (candelas per square meter).
- Assessed using glare indices such as Unified Glare Rating or contrast sensitivity function (CSF) in glare conditions.
- Veiling luminance can range from a few cd/m^2 in low glare to >100 cd/m^2 under intense glare such as sunlight.
- A UGR of:
  - <13 is considered imperceptible
  - 13–19: tolerable
  - 25: uncomfortable

Discomfort Glare is a subjective sensation of annoyance or pain due to bright light even when visual performance is not affected [2].

- Assessed via subjective scales, such as the.
  - De Boer rating scale of 1 to 9:
  - 1 = Unbearable
  - 9 = Just noticeable
  - Glare Rating (GR) or Daylight Glare Probability (DGP).
- DGP < 0.35: Imperceptible
- 0.35–0.40: Perceptible
- 0.40–0.45: Disturbing
- 0.45: Intolerable

M. P. Kelly, *Normal Values in Vision Science*,
https://doi.org/10.1007/978-3-032-18207-4_6

Visual Range is the maximum distance at which an object can be seen/recognized against its background.

- Measured in meters or kilometers, most often in driving or aviation situations
- Related to Michelson contrast, meteorological visibility standards and modulation transfer function (MTF)
- Clear day: 20–50 km
- Foggy/bright conditions: 100 m^{-1} km

Photo-stress Recovery Time is the amount of time required for vision to return to normal after exposure to a bright light source [3, 4].

- Measured in seconds using a controlled light exposure followed by a visual acuity or contrast testing
- Healthy adults: 10–30 s
- Older adults or patients with various ocular diseases: 30–60+ seconds

Chromatic Contrast measures the ability to distinguish between colors which is important with tasks such as recognizing traffic lights [5, 6].

- Measured using color contrast sensitivity tests, CIE color difference formulas (e.g., ΔE).
- Expressed in Just Noticeable Differences (JNDs) or ΔE units.
- ΔE > 2–3 is perceivable by the average observer.
- High chromatic contrast (ΔE > 10) = very distinct colors [7, 8].

Of Related Interest Multispectral and Hyperspectral Imaging Integration Advancements in imaging technologies have led to the development of multispectral and hyperspectral devices capable of capturing light across a broad range of wavelengths, including ultraviolet and infrared spectra. Integrating these devices into wearable systems could allow individuals to perceive a wider spectrum of light.

Smith LA, Johnson MT. Expanding human visual perception through multispectral imaging technologies. Adv Opt Eng. 2024;15(2):89–102. https://doi.org/10.1016/j.aoe.2024.02.005.

References

1. Aslam TM, Haider D, Murray IJ. Principles of disability glare measurement: an ophthalmological perspective. Acta Ophthalmol Scand. 2007;85(4):354–60. https://doi.org/10.1111/j.1600-0420.2006.00860.x.
2. Mainster MA, Turner PL. Glare's causes, consequences, and clinical challenges after a century of ophthalmic study. Am J Ophthalmol. 2012;153(4):587–93. https://doi.org/10.1016/j.ajo.2012.01.008.
3. Malik SRK. Macular function tests with special reference to photostress. Int J Ophthalmol. 1971;19(1):3–8.
4. Margrain TH, Thomson D. Sources of variability in the clinical photostress test. Ophthalmic Physiol Opt. 2002;22(1):61–7. https://doi.org/10.1046/j.1475-1313.2002.00044.x.

5. Kim YJ, Kwon M, Legge GE, Qiao N, Greenberg K, Hu Z. Chromatic and achromatic contrast sensitivity functions in normal adults. Invest Ophthalmol Vis Sci. 2017;58(4):2458–65. https://doi.org/10.1167/iovs.16-21066.
6. Page JW, Dainty C. Differential ageing of chromatic and achromatic visual pathways. Vis Res. 2005;45(14):1759–70. https://doi.org/10.1016/j.visres.2005.01.002.
7. Fong SW, Chirila T, Ingraham HJ. Basic and clinical science course. Section 1: update on general medicine. San Francisco: American Academy of Ophthalmology; 2022–2023.
8. Brar VS. Basic and clinical science course. Section 2: fundamentals and principles of ophthalmology. San Francisco: American Academy of Ophthalmology; 2022–2023.

Chapter 7
Environmental and Physiologic Influences on Ocular Parameters

Various factors can cause transient or chronic variations in normal ocular values. Considering them is essential for interpreting measurements accurately.

Diurnal Variation

- Intraocular Pressure (IOP):
  - Typically highest in the early morning hours (~6–8 a.m.)
  - May vary by 4–6 mmHg over 24 h
  - Influenced by aqueous production and episcleral venous pressure
- Central Corneal Thickness (CCT):
  - Thicker in the morning due to overnight corneal swelling
  - May thin by ~10–20 μm by evening
- Retinal Thickness (especially macula):
  - Slight decrease throughout the day in healthy subjects [1, 2]

Postural Changes

- IOP:
  - Increases in supine position due to increased episcleral venous pressure
  - Can rise by 1–6 mmHg when lying flat [3, 4]
- Optic nerve and choroidal volume:

M. P. Kelly, *Normal Values in Vision Science*,
https://doi.org/10.1007/978-3-032-18207-4_7

- Positional changes can affect optic disc appearance (relevant in glaucoma assessment)

Physical Activity and Exercise

- Aerobic exercise:
  - Temporarily lowers IOP
- Weightlifting or Valsalva maneuvers:
  - Can increase IOP due to elevated venous pressure
- Ocular perfusion pressure may fluctuate depending on systemic blood pressure during and after exercise

Diet and Substances

- Caffeine:
  - May cause mild transient IOP elevation (~1–2 mmHg)
- Alcohol:
  - Can lower IOP transiently
- High-salt intake:
  - May slightly increase IOP in salt-sensitive individuals
- Hydration:
  - Large fluid intake in short time can temporarily increase IOP

Hormonal and Circadian Factors

- Menstrual cycle:
  - Fluctuations in corneal thickness and curvature
- Pregnancy:
  - Tends to lower IOP due to hormonal changes
- Cortisol levels:
  - Circadian pattern mirrors IOP variations

Altitude and Atmospheric Pressure

- High altitude:
  - Mild reduction in IOP due to decreased atmospheric pressure.
  - Possible changes in retinal and choroidal blood flow due to hypoxia.
  - Can increase risk of retinal hemorrhages (esp. in high-altitude retinopathy).

Temperature and Climate

- Cold environments:
  - Vasoconstriction may alter ocular blood flow.
  - Possibly minor reductions in IOP.
- Humidity and dry climates:
  - May affect tear film quality, impacting corneal measurements.

Systemic Physiologic States

- Hypertension:
  - Chronic high BP may elevate IOP.
  - Affects retinal vessel calibers and ocular perfusion.
- Sleep apnea:
  - Associated with fluctuating IOP and risk for normal-tension glaucoma.
- Stress and anxiety:
  - Can transiently raise IOP and blood pressure.

Timing and Repeatability

- Timing of measurement:
  - Always note the time of day when measuring IOP, RNFL, macular thickness.
- Repeat measurements:
  - Diurnal and environmental factors necessitate multiple readings for accurate baselines.

Of Related Interest
Mccafferty and Berdahl's model enables a demonstration of IOP response by glaucoma type with a basic understanding of its mechanistic effects and likewise the probable outcome of treatment combinations. Assignments of independent pharmacologic or surgical outflow and inflow facilities allow prediction of the new interventional IOP responses in any possible combination. The equations enable calculation of the interventional facilities by their IOP responses. In practical terms, the equations facilitate its use in a glaucoma pressure calculator, not unlike an intraocular lens calculator: Intraocular Pressure Equations Utilizing Aqueous Fluid Flow and Flow Facility in the Steady-State and Time-Dependent Domains; McCafferty S, Berdahl J. Intraocular pressure equations utilizing aqueous fluid flow and flow facility in the steady-state and time-dependent domains. Clin Ophthalmol. 2025;19:2901–11. https://doi.org/10.2147/OPTH.S531475

Of Related Interest
Long-duration spaceflight has been associated with a constellation of ocular changes in astronauts including Spaceflight-Associated Neuro-ocular Syndrome (SANS). These changes are believed to result from fluid shifts leading to increased intracranial pressure resulting in ocular alterations including optic disc edema, choroidal folds, and refractive shifts, among others. These changes can persist for months after returning to Earth. The exact pathophysiology remains under investigation.

Further Reading

Lee AG, Mader TH, Gibson CR, Tarver WJ, Rabiei P, Riascos RF, et al. Spaceflight associated neuro-ocular syndrome (SANS) and the neuro-ophthalmologic effects of microgravity: a review and an update. NPJ Microgravity. 2020;6:7.

Svoronos A, Patel NB, Macias BR, Laurie SS, Samuels BC, Stenger MB. Analysis of spaceflight-associated biometric and refractive changes in astronauts. Am J Ophthalmol. 2025;240:1–8.

References

1. David R, Zangwill L, Briscoe D, et al. Diurnal intraocular pressure variations: an analysis of 690 diurnal curves. Br J Ophthalmol. 1992;76(5):280–3. https://doi.org/10.1136/bjo.76.5.280.
2. Kotecha A, White ET, Shewry JM, Garway-Heath DF. The relationship between diurnal variations in intraocular pressure and central corneal thickness. Invest Ophthalmol Vis Sci. 2009;50(9):4309–13. https://doi.org/10.1167/iovs.08-3154.
3. Lam A, Wu YF, Wong LY, Ho NL. IOP variations from sitting to supine postures determined by rebound tonometer. J Optom. 2013;6(2):95–101. https://doi.org/10.1016/j.optom.2013.03.001.
4. Najmanová E, Pluháček F, Haklová M, Faltýnková P, Holá M, Vrána J, et al. Intraocular pressure response affected by changing of sitting and supine positions. Acta Ophthalmol. 2019;97(7):e968–72. https://doi.org/10.1111/aos.14116.

Chapter 8
Ocular Disorders Triggered by Environmental Factors Affecting Normal Vision

Cataracts

Prolonged exposure to ultraviolet (UV-B) radiation, ionizing radiation, smoking.

Cortical cataracts are especially linked to UV exposure [1, 2].

Conjunctivitis (Allergic or Irritant)

Pollen, dust, smoke, industrial chemicals.

Includes seasonal allergic conjunctivitis, vernal conjunctivitis.

Contact Lens-Associated Infections

Contaminated water introducing Acanthamoeba, fungi.

Dry Eye Disease (DED)

Air pollution, low humidity, wind, screen exposure, smoke, and air conditioning [3].

More common in urban and industrial locations.

Fungal Keratitis thrives in hot climates and can have potentially catastrophic visual results. It is caused by the many species of fungi capable of colonizing human tissue [4].

M. P. Kelly, *Normal Values in Vision Science*,
https://doi.org/10.1007/978-3-032-18207-4_8

Ocular Surface Squamous Neoplasia (OSSN)

UV radiation, HPV, HIV co-infection, environmental carcinogens [5].

More common in Africa and areas with high UV exposure.

Photokeratitis

Acute overexposure to UV-B light, especially from snow, water, or welding arcs.

More common in high-altitude, snowy, or marine environments.

Pinguecula

Chronic UV exposure and wind/dust irritation.

Often precedes pterygium.

Pterygium

Chronic UV exposure, dry and dusty climates.

More common in populations living near the equator or bright, sunny environments.

Solar Retinopathy

Direct exposure to sunlight or solar eclipses without eye protection.

Results in damage to photoreceptors and the retinal pigment epithelium.

Trachoma

Repeated infections with *Chlamydia trachomatis*, often spread in areas with poor sanitation, limited water access and high fly populations.

Environmental factors such as dust, crowding, and lack of hygiene play a role in transmission and progression.

Of Related Interest A broad overview of the effects of various environments including urban, domestic, socio-economic, politico-cultural, biotic, and abiotic on eradication of preventable blindness.

Johnson G. The environment and the eye. Eye. 2004;18:1235–50. doi:10.1038/sj.eye.6701369.KEY WORDS: UV radiation, Dry eye, Pterygium, Photokeratitis, Trachoma, Contact lens-associated

References

1. Robman L, Taylor H. External factors in the development of cataract. Eye (Lond). 2005;19(10):1074–82. https://doi.org/10.1038/sj.eye.6701964.
2. MacFarlane ER, Donnelly L, El-Osta A, et al. UV light and the ocular lens: a review of exposure models and relationship to human cortical and nuclear cataract. Front Ophthalmol. 2024;14:1414483. https://doi.org/10.3389/fopht.2024.1414483.
3. Ye J, He J, Wang C, et al. Smoking and risk of age-related cataract: a meta-analysis. Invest Ophthalmol Vis Sci. 2012;53(4):3885–95. https://doi.org/10.1167/iovs.12-9703.
4. Carnt N, Wu Y, Stapleton F, et al. Acanthamoeba keratitis risk factors for daily wear contact lens users: a case-control study. Ophthalmology. 2023;130(1):48–55. https://doi.org/10.1016/j.ophtha.2022.07.018.
5. Alves M, Asbell P, Stapleton F, et al. Impact of environmental conditions on the ocular surface: a systematic review. Ocul Surf. 2023;27:40–61. https://doi.org/10.1016/j.jtos.2023.03.001.

Chapter 9
Biomarkers in Ophthalmology and Vision Science

With recent advancements in noninvasive ophthalmic imaging technologies, including optical coherence tomography (OCT) and optical coherence tomography angiography (OCTA), detection of subclinical disease may be made prior to irreversible damage occurring. Clinical utility of new and existing ophthalmic biomarkers depends heavily on having robust and accurate normal reference values. Without a well-defined baseline, it is difficult to interpret deviations that may indicate pathology. Biomarkers are key in the early diagnosis, disease progression monitoring, and treatment assessment for a range of ophthalmic conditions including age-related macular degeneration, diabetic retinopathy, glaucoma, and keratoconus. These new imaging technologies allow, for example, detection of retinal nerve fiber layer thinning in pre-perimetric glaucoma, offer noninvasive and repeatable ways to monitor disease, and provide systemic disease detection in diabetes and hypertension. Recent research is looking at ocular biomarkers for identifying or predicting systemic risk of cardiovascular disease, multiple sclerosis, Alzheimer's, and others.

Examples of Retinal Biomarkers and Detection Methods

1. Retinal Nerve Fiber Layer (RNFL) Thickness
   - Decreased thickness is associated with glaucoma, multiple sclerosis, and Alzheimer's disease [1–3].
   - Measured using Optical Coherence Tomography (OCT).
2. Ganglion Cell Layer (GCL) and Inner Plexiform Layer (IPL) Thickness
   - Thinning is seen in glaucoma and neurodegenerative diseases.
   - Useful in early detection of cognitive impairment.

M. P. Kelly, *Normal Values in Vision Science*,
https://doi.org/10.1007/978-3-032-18207-4_9

3. Drusen
    - Extracellular deposits characteristic of age-related macular degeneration (AMD).
    - Visible on fundus photography and OCT.
4. Hyperreflective Foci
    - Considered signs of retinal inflammation and degeneration in such diseases as diabetic retinopathy and AMD [4].
5. Retinal Vascular Caliber
    - Changes in arteriolar or venular diameter are associated with hypertension, stroke, and cardiovascular risk.
    - Assessed via retinal imaging (retinal fundus photography).
6. Aβ (Amyloid-beta) Deposition in Retina
    - Suggests a potential early biomarker for Alzheimer's disease.
    - Detected using hyperspectral imaging and fluorescent ligands in research settings.
7. Macular Thickness and Volume
    - Changes can indicate diabetic macular edema, AMD, and retinal vein occlusion.
    - Measured via OCT.
8. Microaneurysms
    - Early sign of diabetic retinopathy.
    - Detected via fluorescein angiography or fundus photography.
9. Retinal Oxygen Saturation
    - Altered levels associated with diabetic retinopathy and glaucoma [5].
    - Measured using retinal oximetry.
10. Electroretinogram (ERG) Parameters
    - Used to assess retinal function, especially in inherited retinal diseases and retinopathies.
    - Reduced amplitudes and delayed implicit times indicate dysfunction.
11. Central Retinal Thickness (CRT)
    - Used to monitor macular edema in diabetic retinopathy, AMD, and retinal vein occlusion.
    - Assessed by OCT; a key parameter in clinical trials for anti-VEGF therapies.
12. Subretinal Fluid (SRF) and Intraretinal Fluid (IRF)
    - Biomarkers for exudative AMD and central serous chorioretinopathy.
    - Quantified by OCT.

13. Choroidal Thickness
    - Changes noted in central serous chorioretinopathy, AMD, and high myopia.
    - Measured using Enhanced Depth Imaging-OCT (EDI-OCT).
14. Retinal Pigment Epithelium (RPE) Alterations
    - RPE atrophy and dysfunction are seen in late-stage AMD and inherited retinal dystrophies.
    - Assessed via fundus autofluorescence and OCT.
15. Vascular Density and Perfusion Metrics (via OCT-Angiography)
    - Reduced capillary density is a hallmark in diabetic retinopathy and glaucoma.
    - Optical Coherence Tomography Angiography (OCT-A) provides noninvasive visualization.
16. Lipofuscin Accumulation
    - Reflects photoreceptor and RPE metabolism; excessive accumulation is toxic.
    - Identified using fundus autofluorescence (FAF); implicated in Stargardt disease and AMD.
17. Cone and Rod Density
    - Decreased in inherited retinal diseases like retinitis pigmentosa.
    - High-resolution adaptive optics scanning laser ophthalmoscopy (AO-SLO) used for measurement.
18. Retinal Blood Flow
    - Altered in diabetic retinopathy, glaucoma, and AMD.
    - Assessed using Doppler OCT, laser speckle flowgraphy, or fluorescein angiography.
19. Neuroinflammatory Markers in Retina
    - Includes cytokines such as TNF-α, IL-6, IL-1β.
    - Elevated in glaucoma, diabetic retinopathy, and optic neuritis.
    - Measured via aqueous/vitreous sampling and immunoassays.
20. Glial Fibrillary Acidic Protein (GFAP) Expression
    - Marker of Müller cell activation and retinal stress.
    - Upregulated in retinal degenerative diseases; detected in histopathology or imaging with specific tracers.

Of Related Interest A new field of study: Oculomics; this term made its first appearance in the scientific literature in February 2020. The publication laid the foundation for the field emphasizing the potential of retinal imaging to reveal biomarkers indicative of systemic health conditions.

Denniston AK, Keane PA, Tufail A. Insights into systemic disease through retinal imaging-based oculomics. Transl Vis Sci Technol. 2020;9(2):6. https://doi.org/10.1167/tvst.9.2.6.

References

1. London A, Benhar I, Schwartz M. The retina as a window to the brain – from eye research to CNS disorders. Nat Rev Neurol. 2013;9(1):44–53. https://doi.org/10.1038/nrneurol.2012.227.
2. den Haan J, Morrema THJ, Verbraak FD, et al. Retinal thickness correlates with parietal cortical atrophy in early-onset Alzheimer's disease and controls. Alzheimers Dement (Amst). 2018;10:49–55. https://doi.org/10.1016/j.dadm.2018.02.002.
3. Abràmoff MD, Fort PE, Han IC, et al. Retinal imaging and biomarkers for Alzheimer's disease. Alzheimers Dement (Amst). 2018;10:196–202. https://doi.org/10.1016/j.dadm.2018.01.003.
4. Tanabe F, Yamada Y, Mizoguchi T, et al. Hyperreflective foci on optical coherence tomography as a predictive factor of visual outcome in diabetic macular edema. Sci Rep. 2020;10:20861. https://doi.org/10.1038/s41598-020-77947-3.
5. Tan O, Li G, Lu AT, et al. Mapping of macular substructures with optical coherence tomography for glaucoma diagnosis. Ophthalmology. 2008;115(6):949–56. https://doi.org/10.1016/j.ophtha.2007.08.056.

Chapter 10
The Ocular Structures

The human eye is composed of intricately organized structures that work in concert to capture, focus, and process visual information. Each structure is specialized for a distinct function, whether it be protection, light refraction, accommodation, or image transmission, all are interdependent.

The *Choroid* is a layer of the eye situated between the retina and the sclera, rich in blood vessels and crucial for providing nutrients to the retina.

Thickness: The choroidal thickness varies depending on the location within the eye. On average, it is approximately 200–300 microns (μm) in thickness. The thickness can be greater in the posterior pole and thinner in the peripheral regions.

Choroidal vascular index (CVI) in a healthy adult has been reported as 65.61% ± 2.33%. CVI is a novel, quantitative imaging biomarker defined as the ratio of vascular area to the total choroidal area and is used to assess choroidal vascular structure and function. It is a parameter derived from optical coherence tomography (OCT) imaging. CVI is calculated by determining the ratio of the area of the choroidal vessels (luminal area) to the total choroidal area [1].

Flow Velocity: Blood flow velocity in the choroid is typically measured using techniques such as Doppler ultrasound or optical coherence tomography (OCT). The mean flow velocity in the choroidal vessels can vary, but average values are in the range of 5–15 cm/s [2].

The *Retina* is light sensitive and is composed of several layers, each with its own characteristics. The retina uses the phototransduction cascade to convert light information into neurochemical signals which are sent to the brain to generate vision.

Retinal Layers

- Nerve Fiber Layer (NFL)
  - Thickness: In the range of 100 microns [3], thinning toward the periphery.

M. P. Kelly, *Normal Values in Vision Science*,
https://doi.org/10.1007/978-3-032-18207-4_10

  - Flow Velocity: Blood flow in the NFL is less frequently measured, but it generally reflects the flow within the retinal vessels supplying this layer.
- Ganglion Cell Complex (GCC)
  - Thickness: Varies and is roughly 80–110 microrons (μm).
  - Flow Velocity: Similar to NFL, the flow velocity in the GCL is indirectly assessed through retinal blood flow measurements.
- Inner Plexiform Layer (IPL)
  - Thickness: Approximately 20–30 microns (μm).
  - Flow Velocity: This layer's flow velocity is also measured indirectly through overall retinal blood flow studies.
- Inner Nuclear Layer (INL)
  - Thickness: Roughly 40–50 microns (μm).
  - Flow Velocity: As with other inner layers, specific flow velocity data is typically derived from retinal blood flow measurements.
- Outer Plexiform Layer (OPL)
  - Thickness: About 10–20 microns (μm).
  - Flow Velocity: Blood flow in the OPL is usually part of general retinal blood flow studies.
  - Flow Velocity: N/A
- Outer Nuclear Layer (ONL)
  - Thickness: Approximately 60–70 microns (μm).
  - Flow Velocity: Blood flow affecting this layer is measured indirectly through broader retinal blood flow techniques.
- Photoreceptor Layer (PRL)
  - Thickness: Around 10–15 microns (μm) for the outer segments of rods and cones.
  - Flow Velocity: The flow velocity impacting this layer is generally part of overall retinal blood flow assessments.
- Retinal Pigment Epithelium (RPE)
  - Thickness: Approximately 10–15 microns (μm).
  - Flow Velocity: Blood flow in the RPE is part of the broader choroidal flow studies.

Flow Velocities

Retinal Blood Flow: The mean blood flow velocity in the retinal vessels is generally around 2–5 cm/s.

Choroidal Blood Flow: The choroidal circulation, which supports the RPE and outer retinal layers, has average flow velocities of around 5–15 cm/s.

These measurements can vary depending on specific conditions and individual factors, and advanced imaging techniques such as Doppler OCT or Laser Doppler Flowmetry are often used for precise measurements.

The *Vitreous Body* is a transparent gel-like substance (>99% water) that fills the space between the lens and the retina and maintains the eyes shape.
Vitreous Volume: The vitreous humor occupies approximately 80% of the eye's total volume. In an adult human eye, this is roughly 4–5 milliliters (mL).
Vitreous Chamber Depth: The depth of the vitreous chamber (from the lens to the retina) is about 16–17 millimeters (mm).

Flow Velocities
The vitreous humor is a gel-like substance and does not have significant flow velocities in the traditional sense as blood or aqueous humor does. However, the vitreous body does exhibit some movement:

Vitreous Flow: While the vitreous humor itself does not flow like a fluid, it does undergo subtle movements due to physiological processes, including vitreous liquefaction and the movement of the eye. These movements are generally slow and not quantified in the same manner as blood flow.
Vitreous Liquefaction: Over time, the vitreous can become more liquid and exhibit slight internal movements. This process is gradual and varies from person to person.

Detailed measurements and flow dynamics are typically assessed using imaging techniques and are more focused on the changes and conditions within the vitreous rather than quantifiable flow velocities.

The *Optic Nerve* is a critical structure responsible for transmitting visual information from the retina to the brain.

- Optic Nerve Diameter
  - Intraocular Portion: The diameter of the optic nerve head (where the nerve exits the eye) is approximately 1.5–2.0 mm.
  - Retrobulbar Portion: The diameter of the optic nerve behind the eye (retrobulbar portion) can be around 3–4 mm.

- Optic Nerve Length
  - The total length of the optic nerve from the eye to the brain is approximately 40–50 mm.

Optic nerve normal cup-to-disc ratio: <0.5.
ON has 1.2–1.5 million axons.

Flow Velocities
- Optic Nerve Blood Flow
  - Mean Flow Velocity: The blood flow velocity in the optic nerve can vary. Typical values are around 10–20 cm/s. This is measured using techniques such as Doppler ultrasound or laser Doppler flowmetry.

Pulsatile Flow: The optic nerve experiences pulsatile blood flow related to the cardiac cycle, with peak velocities occurring with each heartbeat [3].

The *Ciliary body* is a ring-like structure in the eye involved in adjusting the lens for focusing and producing aqueous humor, the fluid that nourishes the eye.

- Ciliary Body Thickness
  - Anterior Portion: Approximately 2–3 mm.
  - Posterior Portion: The thickness can be slightly greater, but specific values can vary among individuals.
- Ciliary Body Length
  - The ciliary body extends about 3–4 mm from the anterior edge of the retina to the scleral spur.
- Ciliary Processes
  - Number: Typically, 70–80 ciliary processes.
  - Height: Each ciliary process is about 1–2 mm in height.

Flow Velocities

- Ciliary Body Blood Flow
  - Mean Flow Velocity: Blood flow velocity in the ciliary body is less commonly measured directly. However, blood flow in the ciliary processes is typically part of overall choroidal blood flow studies.
  - Choroidal Blood Flow: Since the ciliary body is closely associated with the choroidal circulation, its blood flow is often reflected in studies of the choroidal blood flow, which is around 5–15 cm/s.

The *Cornea* is the transparent dome-shaped outer layer that plays a crucial role in focusing light onto the retina and acts as a protective barrier while contributing significantly to refraction.

- Thickness:
  - Central Cornea: Approximately 500–550 microns (μm)
  - Peripheral Cornea: Thinner than the central cornea, around 400–500 μm
- Diameter:
  - Horizontal Diameter: About 11.5–12 mm
  - Vertical Diameter: Approximately 10.5–11 mm

The *Iris* regulates light exposure entering the eye.

- Diameter:
  - Horizontal Diameter: Approximately 11–12 mm
  - Vertical Diameter: Around 9–10 mm
- Thickness:
  - At the Pupil: About 0.5–1 mm
  - At the Periphery: Approximately 1–2 mm

- Flow Velocities:
  - Blood flow in the iris is generally measured indirectly through studies of overall anterior segment blood flow. The velocity of blood flow in the iris can be around 2–5 cm/s.

The *Pupil* is the central opening of the iris that allows light to enter and ultimately reach the retina.

- Diameter:
  - Normal Range: Typically, 2–8 mm, depending on light conditions and individual variation

- Amplitude: up to 0.5 mm, approximately 4% of the iris diameter
- Frequency: 0.1 to 2 oscillations per second

Of Related Interest They present a single case who can change pupil size on command with dilation of pupil diameter of around 0.8 mm, and constriction of around 2.4 mm. Using modern pupillometric and optometric techniques in combination with measuring electrodermal activity, various indirect mechanisms possibly mediating this phenomenon were tested. None of the testing could support an indirect strategy as the mode of action, suggesting direct voluntary control of pupil size in the present case.

Eberhardt LV, Grön G, Ulrich M, Huckauf A, Strauch C. Direct voluntary control of pupil constriction and dilation: Exploratory evidence from pupillometry, optometry, skin conductance, perception, and functional MRI. *Int J Psychophysiol.* 2021;168:33–42. PMID: 34391820. https://doi.org/10.1016/j.ijpsycho.2021.08.001.

The *Lens* is a flexible, transparent structure directly behind the iris which focuses entering light onto the retina.

- Thickness:
  - Central Lens: Approximately 4–5 mm
  - Equatorial Region: Around 3–4 mm [4, 5]

- Diameter:
  - Horizontal Diameter: 9–10 mm
  - Vertical Diameter: 9–10 mm

The *Sclera* is the white, outer layer of the eye that provides the structural support and helps to maintain the eyes shape.

- Thickness:
  - At the Equator: Approximately 0.5–1.0 mm
  - At the Posterior Pole: About 0.7–1.0 mm

- Diameter:
  - Horizontal Diameter: Roughly 24 mm
  - Vertical Diameter: Approximately 23 mm

Eyelids are made of skin that covers and uncovers the eye to spread tears and protect the eye.

- Thickness:
  - Upper Eyelid: Approximately 1–2 mm thick
  - Lower Eyelid: Similar to the upper eyelid, around 1–2 mm thick
- Length:
  - Horizontal Length: Typically, about 28–30 mm from one corner of the eye to the other

Eyelashes are curved follicles along the eyelid edges that provide protection from environmental debris, and enhance sensory input.

- Length:
  - Upper Eyelashes: Typically, 6–12 mm in length.
  - Lower Eyelashes: Generally shorter, around 4–8 mm.
- Density:
  - Upper Eyelash Line: About 90–150 lashes per eye.
  - Lower Eyelash Line: Approximately 70–80 lashes per eye.

The six *Extraocular Muscles* control the movement of the eye.

- Size and Length:
  - Lateral Rectus: 35–40 mm in length
  - Medial Rectus: Similar in length to the lateral rectus, 35–40 mm
  - Superior Rectus: 30–35 mm in length
  - Inferior Rectus: Similar in length to the superior rectus, 30–35 mm
  - Superior Oblique: 25–30 mm in length
  - Inferior Oblique: 25–30 mm in length

References

1. Agrawal R, Gupta P, Tan KA, Cheung CMG, Wong TY, Cheng CY, et al. Choroidal vascularity index in central serous chorioretinopathy. Retina. 2016;36(9):1646–51.
2. Riva CE, Titze P, Hero M, Movaffaghy A, Petrig BL. Choroidal blood flow in the human eye. Prog Retin Eye Res. 2005;24(2):183–203.
3. Budenz DL, Anderson DR, Varma R, Schuman JS, Cantor LB, Savell J, et al. Determinants of normal retinal nerve fiber layer thickness measured by Stratus OCT. Ophthalmology. 2007;114(6):1046–52. https://doi.org/10.1016/j.ophtha.2006.08.046. Erratum in: Ophthalmology. 2008;115(3):472
4. Fong SW, Chirila T, Ingraham HJ. Basic and clinical science course. Section 1: Update on general medicine. San Francisco: American Academy of Ophthalmology; 2022–2023.
5. Brar VS. Basic and Clinical Science Course. Section 2: Fundamentals and principles of ophthalmology. San Francisco: American Academy of Ophthalmology; 2022–2023.

Chapter 11
Visual Function and Ocular Dynamics

Visual function and ocular dynamics encompass the physiological processes that enable the eye to perceive, focus, and respond to visual stimuli. This includes the coordinated actions of accommodation, pupillary reflexes, ocular motility, and the intricate neural pathways that process light into visual perception. Ocular dynamics refer not only to mechanical movements but also to fluid regulation, intraocular pressure maintenance, and the constant interaction between optical structures and neurological control.

Saccades

- Speed:
  - Peak Velocity: Saccades can reach speeds of approximately 300–700 degrees per second (°/s), with the exact speed varying depending on the size of the saccade and the individual.
- Rates:
  - Frequency: Saccades occur at a rate of several per second during tasks such as reading or scanning. The rate can be influenced by the complexity of the visual task and the individual's cognitive load.
  - Amplitude: The distance covered by a saccade varies widely. Small saccades may cover a few degrees, while larger saccades can exceed 30 degrees [1].

M. P. Kelly, *Normal Values in Vision Science*,
https://doi.org/10.1007/978-3-032-18207-4_11

Micro Saccades

- Speed:
  - Peak Velocity: Micro saccades are much slower than regular saccades, with speeds ranging from 10 to 30 degrees per second (°/s).
- Frequency:
  - Micro saccades occur continuously and are present at a rate of 1–2 micro saccades per second. They help stabilize the retinal image and are crucial for visual perception.
- Amplitude:
  - Micro saccades are very small, usually covering less than 1 degree of visual angle [2, 3].

Nystagmus is a neurological condition characterized by involuntary, rhythmic movements of the eyes, which can occur in various directions (horizontal, vertical, or torsional/rotational). These eye movements can be subtle or pronounced and may be unilateral or bilateral. Nystagmus can be congenital or acquired later in life due to a variety of causes, including inner ear disorders, neurological diseases, head trauma, or certain medications. Depending on its type and cause, nystagmus may affect balance, coordination, and vision, often leading to blurred or unstable visual perception.

- Speed:
  - Slow Phase Velocity: During the slow phase of nystagmus, the speed can vary significantly. It typically ranges from 2 to 20 degrees per second (°/s) in various types of nystagmus.
  - Fast Phase Velocity: In those forms of nystagmus with a fast phase, or corrective phase, the velocity can reach speeds of up to 100–200 degrees per second (°/s).
- Rates:
  - Frequency: Nystagmus typically has a frequency of 1–4 cycles per second (Hz). The exact rate depends on the type and cause of the nystagmus.
  - Amplitude: The amplitude of nystagmus can range from a few degrees to more significant angles, depending on the type and underlying cause.

Torsional nystagmus is a type of involuntary eye movement characterized by a rhythmic oscillation of the eyes in a torsional (rotational) direction. Torsional nystagmus can be a symptom of various conditions. While specific measurements can vary from person to person, there are general aspects and parameters that can be considered when assessing torsional nystagmus:

Frequency: The frequency of nystagmus can vary, but it is typically measured in Hertz (Hz), indicating how many cycles of movement occur in one second.

Amplitude: This refers to the extent of eye movement in degrees. Amplitude can be measured by assessing the angle of rotation of the eye during the nystagmus episodes.
Duration: The length of time that the nystagmus lasts can be recorded, which may vary depending on the underlying cause.
Phase: Torsional nystagmus may have a specific phase relationship, such as whether it is predominantly in one direction or if there is a change in direction over time.
Latency: This is the time it takes from the onset of a stimulus, such as a change in position or visual target, to the appearance of nystagmus.
Associated Symptoms: Torsional nystagmus may be associated with other symptoms such as vertigo, imbalance, or visual disturbances. These can be qualitatively assessed but may not have specific numerical values.
Diagnostic Tests: Various tests, such as caloric testing or rotational chair testing, may provide quantitative data on nystagmus characteristics.
Visual Acuity Impact: The effect of nystagmus on visual acuity can also be assessed, though it may vary widely among individuals [4, 5].

Color Vision

Total color blindness is extremely rare with a prevalence of approximately 0.003% of the population; 8% of males and 0.5% of females have some form of red-green color blindness. Deuteranomaly is the most common type, ~5% of males. Congenital color deficiency is usually bilateral and symmetric, non-progressive, most often detected in the first decade or so of life and more common in males. Acquired color vision loss occurs later in life most often due to disease, trauma, age, or medication. Optic neuritis, glaucoma, diabetic retinopathy, and macular degeneration, brain or optic nerve lesions, medications, exposure to heavy metals or solvents, and aging can negatively affect color vision. Gene therapy research is underway and has been successful in dichromatic monkeys, giving them trichromatic vision [6, 7].

Types of Color Vision Deficiencies

Type	Description	Prevalence
Trichromacy	Normal color vision	~92% of males, ~99.5% of females
Deuteranomaly	Reduced green sensitivity	~5% of males
Protanomaly	Reduced red sensitivity	~1% of males
Deuteranopia	No green cones	~1% of males
Protanopia	No red cones	~1% of males
Tritanomaly	Reduced blue sensitivity	<0.01% (both sexes)
Tritanopia	No blue cones	<0.01% (both sexes)
Monochromacy	No color perception	~0.003% (very rare)

Color Vision Tests

Test	Detects	Types detected
Neitz Test	Broad	Protan, Deutan, Tritan
Ishihara Plates	Red-green	Protan, Deutan
Hardy-Rand-Rittler (HRR)	Broad	Protan, Deutan, Tritan
Farnsworth D-15	Mod CVD	Protan, Deutan, Tritan
Farnsworth-Munsell 100 Hue	Full gange	All types
Anomaolscope	Precise match	Protan, Deutan
Cambridge Color	Digital	All types
Lantern	Pass/fail test	Protan, Deutan

Of Related Interest In 2025, researchers at the University of California, Berkeley, unveiled a previously unseen color termed "olo." This discovery was achieved through a novel technique that precisely stimulates individual photoreceptor cells in the human retina. This groundbreaking research may open new avenues in the field of visual neuroscience, may expand our understanding of color perception, holds potential for studying visual processing, and developing therapies for color vision deficiencies.

Fong J, Doyle HK, Wang C, Boehm AE, Herbeck SR, Pandiyan VP, et al. Novel color via stimulation of individual photoreceptors at population scale. Sci Adv. 2025;11(16):eadu1052.

Binocular Vision

Binocular vision refers to the ability of both eyes to work together to provide a single, unified visual perception. This system allows for depth perception, a wide field of view, and the ability to judge distances accurately. Fusion combines the slightly different images from each eye into one coherent image, aligning them to avoid double vision. Stereopsis is the ability to perceive depth and three-dimensional structure based on the slightly different images received by each eye.

Methods used in evaluating binocular vision:

- Distance chart: A clinician observes the patient's eyes while they read down a distance chart, looking for when one eye breaks away.
- Bagolini Lenses.
- Lang Test.
- Titmus Test.
- TNO Test.
- Cover Test, Maddox Rod Test.
- Prisms: A 20 diopter base-out prism can be placed in front of one eye while a penlight is shined to check for fusion.

Ocular Tracking Speed

The speed at which the adult human eye can detect moving targets depends on the type of movement and the conditions:

- Smooth Pursuit: This type of tracking is used for following a moving object smoothly. It is effective up to speeds of around 30–60 degrees per second (°/s). Beyond this range, tracking becomes less accurate, and saccades are often used to refocus.
- Static Detection: In bright light conditions, the human eye can detect movements as slow as 0.1 degrees per second (°/s).
- Dynamic Vision: For high-speed tracking and detection, the eye can effectively perceive movements up to around 60–100 degrees per second (°/s) under normal conditions. This range allows for the detection of objects moving quickly across the visual field.

These factors help in understanding how the human visual system processes and responds to visual stimuli in different lighting conditions and movement scenarios.

Lowest Level of Luminance Recognition

The lowest level of luminance recognition is the minimum light level at which the human eye can detect and perceive objects.

- Scotopic Vision: Under very low light conditions (dark adaptation), the human eye can detect light levels as low as about 10^{-6} to 10^{-7} lux. This is typically achieved under dark-adapted conditions where rod cells are predominantly responsible for vision.

Of Related Interest Near-infrared spatiotemporal Color Vision in Humans Enabled by Up-conversion Contact Lenses introduces the potential of wearable polymeric materials for noninvasive NIR vision assisting humans in perceiving and transmitting temporal, spatial, and color dimensions of near-infrared light. https://doi.org/10.1016/j.cell.2025.04.019

References

1. Leigh RJ, Zee DS. Saccades. In: The neurology of eye movements. 5th ed. New York: Oxford University Press; 2015. p. 1–45.
2. Engbert R, Kliegl R. Microsaccades uncover the orientation of covert attention. Vision Res. 2003;43(9):1035–45. https://doi.org/10.1016/S0042-6989(03)00044-1.
3. Martinez-Conde S, Macknik SL, Hubel DH. The role of fixational eye movements in visual perception. Nat Rev Neurosci. 2004;5(3):229–40. https://doi.org/10.1038/nrn1341.

4. Abadi RV, Bjerre A, McLeod D. Motor and sensory characteristics of infantile nystagmus. Brain. 2002;125(9):1858–68. https://doi.org/10.1093/brain/awf195.
5. Shaikh AG, Zee DS. Gaze fixation deficits and their implication in ataxia. Ann Neurol. 2009;65(1):71–80. https://doi.org/10.1002/ana.21676.
6. Kingma H, Stegeman P, Vogels R. Ocular torsion induced by static and dynamic visual stimulation and static whole body roll. Eur Arch Otorhinolaryngol. 1997;254(Suppl 1):S61–3. https://doi.org/10.1007/BF02439726.
7. Groen E, Bos JE, de Graaf B. Contribution of the otoliths to the human torsional vestibulo-ocular reflex. J Vestib Res. 1999;9(1):27–36.

Chapter 12
Fluids in the Human Eye

The eye is a complex organ that involves fluid mechanics in several key processes, particularly in the management of intraocular fluid and the maintenance of intraocular pressure. The fluid mechanics of the human eye are critical for its function and health. Understanding the normative measurements of flow velocities, intraocular pressure, and other parameters is essential for diagnosing and managing ocular conditions, including glaucoma. Advanced imaging and measurement techniques continue to enhance our understanding of these processes.

Aqueous Humor Dynamics

- Production: The aqueous humor is produced by the ciliary body, primarily in the posterior chamber of the eye.
- Flow Path: The aqueous humor flows from the posterior chamber through the pupil into the anterior chamber and exits through the trabecular meshwork into Schlemm's canal.
- Normative Measurements:
    - Production Rate: The aqueous humor is produced at a rate of approximately 2–3 microliters per minute.
    - Intraocular Pressure (IOP): Normative IOP values range from 10 to 21 mmHg, with an average of about 15 mmHg. The IOP is a critical parameter in assessing eye health, particularly in glaucoma.

M. P. Kelly, *Normal Values in Vision Science*,
https://doi.org/10.1007/978-3-032-18207-4_12

Flow Velocities

- Flow Velocity: The flow velocity of the aqueous humor can vary based on several factors, including intraocular pressure and the resistance of the outflow pathways. Typical velocities in the anterior chamber can range from 0.1 to 0.5 mm/s for the flow of aqueous humor.

Outflow Resistance

- Trabecular Meshwork: This structure provides resistance to the outflow of aqueous humor. Increased resistance can lead to elevated IOP, a key factor in glaucoma.
- Normative Measurements:
  - Outflow can be estimated to be around 0.2 to 0.3 μL/min/mmHg in healthy individuals [1–3].

Vitreous Humor

- Composition and Flow: The vitreous humor is a gel-like substance that fills the space between the lens and the retina. While it is not actively circulating like aqueous humor, its mechanical properties and viscosity influence the overall fluid dynamics within the eye.
- Viscosity: The viscosity of vitreous humor is significantly higher than that of aqueous humor, impacting the movement of cells and other substances [4, 5].

Retinal Blood Flow

- Blood Supply: The retina receives its blood supply mainly from the central retinal artery and choroidal circulation. The fluid mechanics of blood flow in these vessels is crucial for maintaining retinal health.
- Normative Measurements: Retinal blood flow values are approximately 40–60 mL/100 g/min, although measurements can vary based on individual factors [6, 7].

Vitreous Humor: Particulates in the vitreous are measured by size, concentration, molecular composition, and morphology using techniques such as flow cytometry, OCT, microscopy, PCR, and mass spectrometry.

- Cells: 5–30 microns
- Exosomes: 30–150 nm
- DNA/RNA: 100 bp to several kb
- Glucose: 50–75 mg/dL
- RPE cells: 10–20 microns

Aqueous Humor: Contains fewer cells, but inflammatory cells may appear in response to infection, inflammation, or tumors. Methods including flow cytometry, confocal microscopy, and slit-lamp biomicroscopy are used for analysis [8, 9].

- Exosomes: 30–150 nm
- Glucose: 50–75 mg/dL

Tears: Contain proteins, lipids, cells, and molecular markers, analyzed similarly to other ocular fluids.

Other Fluids:

- Ciliary Body Fluid: Contributes to aqueous humor and IOP regulation.
- Ocular Lymphatic Fluid: Emerging area of research on lymphatic drainage from the eye, especially the retina.
- Perilymph: Found in the inner ear, relevant to eye movement and balance.
- Subretinal Fluid: Between the retina and RPE, monitored with OCT for retinal conditions.
- Chamber-Adjacent Fluids: Aqueous humor in anterior and posterior chambers are crucial for IOP regulation [10, 11].

Of Related Interest For information on foundational fluid mechanics principles and their biomedical applications:

- Fung YC. Biomechanics: Circulation. 2nd ed. Springer; 1997. doi:10.1007/978-1-4757-2696-1.
- Lupardi E, Cassiano A, Moramarco A, et al. In vitro flow properties of Preserflo Microshunt with an intraluminal stent. Eye. 2025. doi:10.1038/s41433-025-03870-7.

Of Related Interest Human ocular fluid outflow on-chip reveals trabecular meshwork-mediated Schlemm's canal endothelial dysfunction in steroid-induced glaucoma.

Lu R, Kolarzyk AM, Stamer WD, et al. Human ocular fluid outflow on-chip reveals trabecular meshwork-mediated Schlemm's canal endothelial dysfunction in steroid-induced glaucoma. Nat Cardiovasc Res. 2025. https://doi.org/10.1038/s44161-025-00704-3

References

1. Sunderland DK. Aqueous humor circulation. In: StatPearls [Internet]. Treasure Island: StatPearls Publishing; 2023. [cited 2025 Aug 20]. Available from: https://www.ncbi.nlm.nih.gov/books/NBK553209/.
2. Yang MJ. Aqueous humor production and dynamics. In: University of Utah Moran Core; 2022. [cited 2025 Aug 20]. Available from: https://morancore.utah.edu/section-10-glaucoma/aqueous-humor-production-and-dynamics/morancore.utah.edu+1.
3. Toris CB. Measuring the outflow of aqueous humor. Glaucoma Today; 2007. [cited 2025 Aug 20]; Available from: https://glaucomatoday.com/pdfs/GT0907_01.pdfGlaucoma Today
4. Mishra D, et al. Vitreous humor: Composition, characteristics, and clinical implications. J Ocul Biol Dis Infor. 2023;16(1):1–10. Available from: https://www.tandfonline.com/doi/full/10.1080/02713683.2022.2119254Taylor & Francis Online
5. Srikantha N, et al. Determining vitreous viscosity using fluorescence recovery after photobleaching. PLoS One. 2022;17(8):e0269029. Available from: https://journals.plos.org/plosone/article?id=10.1371/journal.pone.0269029PubMed Central
6. Zhang Y, et al. Blood flow MRI of the human retina/choroid during rest and visual stimulation. Invest Ophthalmol Vis Sci. 2012;53(3):1270–6. Available from: https://iovs.arvojournals.org/article.aspx?articleid=2130016IOVS+1
7. Chen Y, et al. Blood flow perfusion in the visual pathway detected by arterial spin labeling MRI. Front Neurosci. 2023;17:104. Available from: https://www.frontiersin.org/articles/10.3389/fnins.2023.1070044/fullPubMed Central
8. Zhan X, et al. Mass spectrometry analysis of human tear fluid biomarkers. J Proteome Res. 2021;20(3):1379–88. Available from: https://pubs.acs.org/doi/10.1021/acs.jproteome.0c00892PubMed Central
9. Shirane M, et al. Current understanding of ocular fluid analysis in uveitis. Transl J Ophthalmol. 2025;3(1):4–10. Available from: https://journals.lww.com/tjop/fulltext/2025/04000/current_understanding_of_ocular_fluid_analysis_in.4.aspxLippincottJournals+1
10. Machiele R, et al. Intraocular pressure. In: StatPearls [Internet]. Treasure Island: StatPearls Publishing; 2024. [cited 2025 Aug 20]. Available from: https://www.ncbi.nlm.nih.gov/books/NBK532237/NCBI.
11. American Academy of Ophthalmology. Eye pressure testing. Eye Health Tips. 2025; [cited 2025 Aug 20]. Available from: https://www.aao.org/eye-health/tips-prevention/eye-pressure-testingAAO

Chapter 13
Applied Measurement Values in Ophthalmic Research by Subspecialty

In the field of *Retina Research*, measurements, velocities, etc., pertain to various aspects of retinal anatomy and function. Current retina research interests include optogenetics and retinal prosthetics, novel drug delivery systems, stem cell therapy and retina regeneration, gene therapy, and artificial intelligence in retinal imaging.

Retinal Layers

- Thickness: The thickness of retinal layers varies by region:
- Fovea (Central Retina): The retinal thickness is about 200–250 μm [1].
- Peripheral Retina: Thicker than the central retina.

Retinal Blood Flow

- Mean Flow Velocity:
- Retinal Vessels: Blood flow velocity in the central retinal artery and vein typically ranges from 2 to 5 centimeters per second (cm/s) [2].
- Choroidal Circulation: The choroidal blood flow velocity, which also affects the outer retinal layers, generally ranges from 5 to 15 cm/s [3].
  And the choroidal vascular index (CVI) in healthy persons has been reported as 65.61% ± 2.33% in healthy people [4].
- Pulsatile Flow: Blood flow in the retina exhibits pulsatility related to the cardiac cycle, with peak velocities corresponding to heartbeats.

Retinal Response and Activation

- Electrophysiological Measurements:
- Visual Evoked Potentials (VEP): These measure the electrical response of the brain to visual stimuli, reflecting the activity of the retina and visual pathways.
- Retinal Imaging:
- Optical Coherence Tomography (OCT): Provides high-resolution images of retinal layers with thickness measurements in microns. This technique helps assess retinal structure and detect abnormalities.

M. P. Kelly, *Normal Values in Vision Science*,
https://doi.org/10.1007/978-3-032-18207-4_13

Retinal Scanning and Tracking

- Saccadic Movements:
- Velocity: Retinal saccadic movements can reach speeds of 300–700 degrees per second (°/s), which impacts how quickly the retina can reorient and process visual information.
- Micro saccades:
- Velocity: Micro saccades have peak velocities of about 10–30 degrees per second (°/s) and occur continuously to stabilize the retinal image [5].

Retinal Sensitivity

- Luminance Detection:
- Lowest Level: The retina can detect light levels as low as 10^{-6} to 10^{-7} lux under scotopic (low light) conditions, where rod photoreceptors are most active [6].

Retinal Diseases and Changes

- Retinal Degeneration: Measurements often involve assessing the thickness of retinal layers and changes in blood flow or response times to understand the extent of retinal diseases such as age-related macular degeneration (AMD) or diabetic retinopathy.

In *Glaucoma Research*, several measurements are critical for diagnosing and monitoring the condition. Glaucoma is a group of eye diseases characterized by damage to the optic nerve, often associated with elevated intraocular pressure (IOP). Much work is being done using OCT imaging to evaluate NFL and ganglion cell layer loss in glaucoma progression. Current research interests include genetics and personalized medicine, neuroprotection and regenerative therapies, improved diagnostic imaging, molecular mechanisms and intraocular press regulation, drug delivery systems and long-acting medications. Some groups are studying OCTA and fractal analysis, a sophisticated way to evaluate the microvascular networks and can capture subtle alterations in the network such as reductions in branching complexity or loss of finer vessels which may be indicators of early glaucoma progression.

Intraocular Pressure (IOP)

- Measurement:
- Normal Range: Typically, 10–21 mmHg (millimeters of mercury).
- Techniques: Measured using tonometry, such as Goldmann applanation tonometry or non-contact tonometry.

Optic Nerve Head (ONH) Parameters

- Disc Cupping
- Cup-to-Disc Ratio
- Optic Nerve Head (ONH) Thickness:
- Average Thickness: Typically ranges around 500–600 microns (μm) but varies with individual factors and disease progression.

Retinal Nerve Fiber Layer (RNFL)

- Thickness:
- Normal Range: Generally, 92.9 ± 9.4 μm [7] in healthy individuals. Thinning of the RNFL is indicative of glaucoma.
- Measurement Techniques:
- Optical Coherence Tomography (OCT): Provides detailed images of RNFL thickness and can detect glaucomatous changes.

Ganglion Cell Complex (GCC)

- Thickness:
- Normal Range: Caries roughly between 80 and 110 (μm). Glaucoma often leads to thinning of the GCC (thickness differs due to age, sex, race, axial length, device used, segmentation applied, etc.)
- Measurement Techniques:
- OCT: Assesses the thickness of the GCC and provides insights into glaucomatous damage.

Visual Field Testing

- Standard Automated Perimetry:
- Detection: Assesses the visual field for defects. Common measures include mean deviation (MD) and pattern standard deviation (PSD).
- Sensitivity:
- Normal Sensitivity: Typically ranges around 1–2 decibels (dB) in a healthy visual field. Glaucoma can reduce sensitivity in specific areas of the visual field.

Ciliary Body and Trabecular Meshwork

- Outflow Facility:
- Measurement: Assessed through techniques such as tonography. Measures the ability of the eye to drain aqueous humor, which affects IOP.

Blood Flow in the Optic Nerve

- Measurement:
- Mean Velocity: Blood flow in the optic nerve head can be measured using Doppler OCT or laser Doppler flowmetry. Normal flow velocities are around 10–20 cm/s. Reduced blood flow can be associated with glaucomatous damage.

Ocular Pulse Amplitude

- Measurement:
- Normal Range: Ocular pulse amplitude (OPA) reflects the pulsatile nature of blood flow in the eye. Altered OPA can be indicative of glaucoma.

Rate of Disease Progression

- Monitoring:
- Longitudinal Changes: Regular monitoring of RNFL, ONH, and visual field over time helps in assessing the rate of disease progression.

Of Related Interest A retrospective case-control analysis was performed on patients with glaucoma and control participants who underwent swept-source optical coherence tomography (SS-OCT) at a single institution. Fujimoto et al. found that eyes with glaucoma had a significantly reduced number of peripapillary perforating scleral vessels compared with healthy controls, independent of age. This reduction may reflect impaired perfusion of the retina and optic nerve suggesting that PPSV count could serve as a novel biomarker for glaucoma risk detection.

Fujimoto S, Maruyama K, Nishida T, et al. Comparison of the number of peripapillary perforating scleral vessels between glaucomatous eyes and healthy eyes. Sci Rep. 2025;15:31459. https://doi.org/10.1038/s41598-025-16480-w

In *Cornea Research*, various measurements are essential for diagnosing, monitoring, and understanding corneal health and diseases. Recent work has been done showing possible corneal endothelial cell morphology with neurodegeneration in mild cognitive impairment and dementia using corneal confocal microscopy. Emerging interests in cornea research include corneal regeneration and stem cell therapy, gene therapy, corneal biomechanics and disease mechanisms, innovative drug delivery systems, and advances in corneal transplantation techniques.

Corneal Thickness

- Central Corneal Thickness (CCT):
- Normal Range: Approximately 500–550 microns (μm).
- Measurement Techniques: Measured using pachymetry (e.g., ultrasonic pachymetry, optical coherence tomography (OCT).)
- Peripheral Corneal Thickness:
- Range: Slightly thicker than the central cornea, often ranging from 550 to 600 μm.

Corneal Curvature

- Keratometry:
- Measurement: Evaluates the curvature of the corneal surface.
- Normal Range: Typically, 7.6–8.6 mm for the radius of curvature, corresponding to about 40–45 diopters (D) in refractive power.
- Topography:
- Techniques: Corneal topography maps the surface curvature and detects irregularities. Measurements include the steepest and flattest meridians.

Corneal Endothelial Cell Density

- Measurement:
- Normal Range: Typically, 2500–3000 cells per square millimeter (cells/mm^2).
- Techniques: Measured using specular microscopy or confocal microscopy.

Corneal Epithelial Thickness

- Measurement:
- Normal Range: Generally, 50–60 microns (μm) at the central cornea.
- Techniques: Assessed using OCT.

Corneal Hysteresis

- Measurement:
- Normal Range: Typically, 8–12 millimeters of mercury (mmHg).

- Techniques: Measured using ocular response analyzer (ORA). Corneal hysteresis reflects the cornea's biomechanical properties and can be indicative of glaucoma risk.

Corneal Topography and Mapping
- Measurements:
- Maps: Provide detailed maps of corneal curvature, elevation, and thickness.
- Techniques: Corneal topography systems, such as those using Placido disks or Scheimpflug imaging.

Corneal Tear Film Stability
- Tear Break-Up Time (TBUT):
- Measurement: The time it takes for the tear film to break up after a blink.
- Normal Range: Typically, greater than 10 s. Shorter times may indicate dry eye disease.

Corneal Velocity and Movement
- Corneal Endothelial Cell Movement:
- Measurement: The movement and density of endothelial cells can be assessed, particularly in diseases affecting cell health.

Corneal Biomechanics
- Measurement Techniques:
- Corneal Deformation Response: Measured using devices such as the Corvis ST, which assesses the cornea's response to air-puff induced deformation.

Corneal Refractive Index
- Measurement:
- Normal Range: Typically, around 1.376.
- Techniques: Refractometry and topography can assess changes in the refractive index due to corneal conditions [8].

Of Related Interest International Ophthalmology published a paper in 2025 that shows a thicker central cornea was associated with thicker corneal epithelium, smaller anterior chamber angle, greater optic nerve sheath diameter, and higher intraocular pressure readings.

Yener AÜ, Özdemir Yıldız Z, Çöllüoğlu Hamurcu Z, et al. The association of corneal thickness with ocular structures from corneal epithelium to optic nerve sheath diameter. Int Ophthalmol. 2025;45:306. https://doi.org/10.1007/s10792-025-03683-3.

In *Neuro-Ophthalmology Research*, values pertain to various aspects of the visual and neurological systems, focusing on the interaction between the eyes and the brain. Fixational eye movements (FEMs) may play a role in enhancing visual acuity, as well as perceptual learning and adaptation; they may have applications in future artificial vision system development. Current research being explored include optic nerve regeneration and neuroprotection, neuro-ophthalmic manifestations of systemic diseases, multiple sclerosis and the optic nerve, and artificial intelligence (AI) in visual pathway disorders.

Of Related Interest Vision requires eye movements, yet our eyes also have miniscule unconscious movements that can blur out fine visual details. Previous work has suggested these small movements aid fine detail perception. This paper investigates this paradox to uncover in which contexts small eye movements help or harm visual acuity. The results indicate that perception is active even at the level of very fine eye movements. https://doi.org/10.1073/pnas.2416266122. 2025

Visual Evoked Potentials (VEPs)
- Latency:
- Prolongation can indicate pathology along the afferent visual pathway.
- Amplitude:
- Normal Range: Amplitude of VEPs is measured in microvolts (μV). Abnormalities can suggest issues with visual pathways or processing.

Ocular Motor Function
- Saccadic Movements:
- Speed: Saccades can reach speeds of 300–700 degrees per second (°/s). Abnormalities in speed or accuracy can indicate neurological disorders.
- Smooth Pursuit:
- Speed: Effective smooth pursuit is up to 30–60 degrees per second (°/s). Difficulty in tracking moving targets may suggest neurological issues.
- Nystagmus:
- Frequency: The frequency of nystagmus typically ranges from 1 to 4 cycles per second (Hz). The velocity and amplitude of the slow phase and (when present) fast phase can indicate different types of nystagmus.

Pupillary Responses
- Pupillary Light Reflex:
- Latency: The reflex typically occurs within 200–300 milliseconds (ms) after exposure to light.
- Pupil Size:
- Normal Range: Typically, 2–8 millimeters (mm) depending on light conditions and individual variation.

Visual Field Testing
- Standard Automated Perimetry:
- Sensitivity: Normal sensitivity in various visual field locations. Reduced sensitivity can indicate damage to visual pathways or cortical areas.
- Field Defects:
- Detection: Scanning for and measuring the extent of visual field defects, which can be indicative of neurological conditions affecting the visual pathways.

Optical Coherence Tomography (OCT)
- Retinal Nerve Fiber Layer (RNFL) Thickness:

- Normal Range: Roughly, 90–110 microns (μm) depending on the instrument used. Thinning can suggest optic nerve damage, often seen in glaucoma or neuro-ophthalmologic disorders.
- Ganglion Cell Complex (GCC) Thickness:
- Normal Range: About roughly 80–110 microns (μm). (Thickness differs due to age, sex, race, axial length, device used, segmentation applied, etc.). Abnormalities can indicate neuro-ophthalmologic conditions [9].

Imaging Techniques
- Magnetic Resonance Imaging (MRI):
- Resolution: MRI provides detailed images of the brain and optic nerves, assessing for structural abnormalities and lesions.
- Computed Tomography (CT):
- Resolution: CT scans help in evaluating acute conditions or bony structures around the eyes and brain.

Visual Pathway Assessment
- Visual Pathway Integrity:
- Assessment: Using various neuroimaging techniques and visual tests to evaluate the health and function of the optic nerve and visual cortex.

Ocular Blood Flow
- Blood Flow Velocity:
- Measurement: Techniques such as Doppler OCT or laser Doppler flowmetry can measure blood flow velocity in the optic nerve head. Normal values typically range around 10–20 cm/s.

Neuro-ophthalmic Symptoms
- Measurement of Symptoms:
- Assessment: Evaluating symptoms such as diplopia (double vision), visual field loss, or eye movement abnormalities, which can provide insights into neurological disorders.

In *Ocular Oncology Research*, measurements and techniques are crucial for diagnosing, monitoring, and treating ocular tumors. Current areas of research interest in ocular oncology include immunotherapy and targeted therapies, gene therapy for inherited retinal tumors, noninvasive diagnostic tools, genomics, and personalized medicine.

Tumor Size and Dimensions
- Measurement:
- Tumor Diameter: Measured in millimeters (mm) using imaging techniques. For example:
- Retinoblastoma: Tumors typically range from 10 to 30 mm in diameter.
- Choroidal Melanoma: Tumors can be up to 20 mm in diameter or more.
- Techniques:
- Ultrasound: Provides measurements of tumor size, thickness, and extent.

- Optical Coherence Tomography (OCT): Offers cross-sectional images to assess tumor dimensions and retinal involvement.
- Magnetic Resonance Imaging (MRI) and Computed Tomography (CT): Used for detailed imaging and precise measurements of the tumor and surrounding structures.

Tumor Growth Rate
- Measurement:
- Growth Rate: Monitored over time to assess how quickly a tumor is growing. This is calculated by comparing tumor size at different time points.
- Techniques:
- Imaging: Serial imaging studies (e.g., ultrasound, MRI) are used to track changes in tumor size and volume.

Tumor Vascularization
- Measurement:
- Blood Flow: Assessing the extent of vascularization within the tumor can help in understanding its aggressiveness and potential for metastasis.
- Techniques:
- Doppler Ultrasound: Measures blood flow within the tumor.
- OCT Angiography: Provides detailed images of blood vessels in the tumor.

Intraocular Pressure (IOP)
- Measurement:
- Normal Range: Typically, 10–21 mmHg. Elevated IOP can be associated with intraocular tumors such as melanoma.
- Techniques:
- Tonometry: Measures the pressure inside the eye, which can be affected by the presence of a tumor.

Tumor Thickness and Extent
- Measurement:
- Thickness: The depth of the tumor can be critical in assessing its stage and potential for treatment.
- Extent: The involvement of surrounding tissues and structures.
- Techniques:
- Ultrasound: Measures tumor thickness and depth.
- MRI: Assesses tumor extent and its relationship with surrounding ocular structures.

Histopathological Evaluation
- Measurement:
- Cell Type and Grade: Determines the type of tumor cells and their grade, which affects prognosis and treatment.
- Techniques:
- Biopsy: A sample of tumor tissue is examined microscopically to determine the cancer type and grade.

Treatment Response
- Measurement:
- Response Assessment: Evaluates how well the tumor responds to treatment. Measurements include changes in tumor size and symptoms.
- Techniques:
- Imaging: Regular follow-up imaging to assess response to therapy.
- Functional Tests: Assessing visual function and other related parameters.

Systemic Spread
- Measurement:
- Metastasis: Checking for spread to other parts of the body, which can be assessed through imaging and blood tests.
- Techniques:
- Whole-Body Imaging: MRI, CT scans, and PET scans to detect metastases [10].

In *Oculoplastic Research*, which focuses on the surgical and medical management of conditions affecting the eyelids, orbit, and surrounding structures, several key measurements and parameters are pertinent. These measurements help in diagnosing conditions, planning surgeries, and assessing outcomes.

Eyelid Measurements
- Eyelid Position and Function:
- Palpebral Fissure: The vertical distance between the upper and lower eyelid margins. Normal range is about 8–11 mm.
- Margin-to-Margin Distance: Measures the distance between the upper and lower eyelid margins. Normal is 9–11 mm.
- Eyelid Tarsal Height:
- Normal Range: Typically, 6–8 mm for the upper eyelid tarsal height.
- Lid Crease Position:
- Normal Range: The position of the eyelid crease varies by individual, but it's typically around 8–10 mm above the upper eyelid margin in females; 6–8 mm in males.

Eyelid Function
- Blink Rate:
- Normal Rate: Typically, 12–15 blinks per minute. Abnormalities can indicate dysfunction.
- Blink Velocity:
- Normal Velocity: Rapid, with typical blink speeds around 200–300 milliseconds (ms) per blink.
- Tear Film Break-Up Time (TBUT):
- Normal Range: Greater than 10 s. Shorter times can indicate dry eye conditions related to tear film instability.

Orbital Measurements
- Orbital Volume: about 30 cm^3
- Measurement: Assessed using imaging techniques such as MRI or CT to evaluate conditions such as orbital tumors or inflammation.

- Orbital Rim Dimensions: 35 mm in height and 45 mm in width. In adults, the depth of the orbit varies from 40 to 45 mm from the orbital entrance to the orbital apex depending on sex and race.
- Measurement: Analyzed using imaging to assess for fractures or other orbital anomalies.

Fat Prolapse and Enophthalmos

- Fat Prolapse:
- Measurement: Evaluated via clinical examination and imaging. Notable in conditions such as orbital septum laxity.
- Enophthalmos:
- Measurement: The degree of posterior displacement of the eye. Measured using imaging or clinical examination, typically noted as a reduction in the eye's projection from the orbital rim by exophthalmometry or Worm's eye view evaluation.

Eyelid Margin Evaluation

- Palpebral Fissure: Vertical distance between the upper and lower eyelid margins.
- Measurement: Normal length is about 8–11 mm. Assessments are important in cases of eyelid malposition such as ectropion or entropion.
- Lid Margin Position:
- Measurement: Important for evaluating conditions such as lid retraction. Measured by margin to reflex distance from corneal light reflex to the upper (MRD1) or lower (MRD2) eyelid margin. Normal MRD1 is 4–5 mm.

Post-Surgical Assessment

- Surgical Outcome Measurements:
- Symmetry: Assessing the symmetry of eyelid position and function post-surgery.
- Healing: Monitoring wound healing and any postoperative complications.

Imaging Techniques

- CT and MRI:
- Measurements: Provide detailed images of the orbit, eyelids, and surrounding tissues. Used to assess conditions such as orbital fractures, tumors, and inflammatory diseases. CT is best for bone evaluation, MRI is best for soft tissues.
- Ultrasound:
- Measurement: Used to evaluate orbital masses and other soft tissue conditions.

Functional Assessments

- Visual Field Testing:
- Measurement: Important for assessing any impact on vision due to eyelid or orbital conditions.
- Eyelid Force Measurement [11]

In *Pediatric Ophthalmology Research*, values are essential for diagnosing, managing, and understanding eye conditions in children.

Visual Acuity

- Measurement:
- Visual Acuity (VA): Assessed using age-appropriate charts or devices. For infants, VA might be estimated using preferential looking tests or visual evoked potentials (VEP).
- Normal Range:
- Infants: VA is typically around 20/400 at birth and improves to approximately 20/25 to 20/40 by age 5–7 years.

Refractive Errors

- Measurement:
- Refraction: Determined using cycloplegic refraction (dilated pupil) to assess for conditions such as myopia, hyperopia, and astigmatism.
- Normal Ranges:
- Infants: +0.50 to +4.00 diopters at birth with refraction being dynamic in infancy as the infant eye is in a constant state of development.

Ocular Motility

- Eye Movements:
- Saccadic Movements: Peak velocities are typically 300–600 degrees per second (°/s). Abnormalities can indicate neurological or developmental issues.
- Smooth Pursuit:
- Speed: Normal pursuit speeds are up to 30–50 degrees per second (°/s). Poor smooth pursuit can be associated with developmental or neurological disorders.
- Nystagmus:
- Frequency: Nystagmus frequencies can range from 1 to 5 cycles per second (Hz). Pediatric nystagmus may be congenital or acquired.

Binocular Vision and Stereopsis

- Measurement:
- Stereopsis: Assessed using tests such as the Randot or Titmus test. Normal stereopsis typically measures in the range of 40–60 arcseconds.
- Binocular Function:
- Cover Test: Evaluates alignment and detects conditions such as strabismus. Measurements include deviation angles in prism diopters (PD).

Ocular Anatomy

- Corneal Diameter:
- Measurement: Typically, 10–12 millimeters (mm) in children.
- Axial Length:
- Measurement: The length of the eye from the front to the back, typically measured in millimeters (mm). Normal axial length is approximately 22–24 mm in children.

Intraocular Pressure (IOP)

- Measurement:
- Normal Range: Typically, 10–18 mmHg in children. Elevated IOP can be a sign of conditions such as congenital glaucoma.
- Techniques:
- Tonometry: Methods include applanation or non-contact tonometry adapted for pediatric use.

Retinal Imaging

- Optical Coherence Tomography (OCT):
- Measurement: Assesses retinal layer thickness and structure. Normal values for retinal thickness vary by age and developmental stage.
- Fundus Photography:
- Measurement: Captures images of the retina for evaluating conditions such as retinopathy of prematurity (ROP) or congenital retinal diseases.

Visual Field Testing

- Measurement:
- Testing: Performed using age-appropriate methods such as automated perimetry for older children or behavioral tests for younger children.

Developmental Milestones

- Visual Development:
- Milestones: Assessing visual skills development at various ages, such as tracking objects, depth perception, and color vision.

Genetic and Systemic Assessments

- Measurement:
- Genetic Testing: For inherited ocular conditions. Measurements include identifying genetic mutations associated with conditions such as Leber congenital amaurosis or retinitis pigmentosa.
- Systemic Conditions:
- Monitoring: Assessing the impact of systemic diseases (e.g., neurofibromatosis) on ocular health.

In *Pediatric Glaucoma Research*, specific measurements and parameters are critical for diagnosing, monitoring, and managing glaucoma in children. Pediatric glaucoma can present differently compared to adults, and understanding these nuances is crucial.

Intraocular Pressure (IOP)

- Measurement:
- Normal Range: Typically, 10–15 mmHg in newborns. Most children with glaucoma will have an IOP higher than 22 mmHg.
- Techniques: Tonometry methods such as Perkins applanation tonometer, non-contact tonometry, or rebound tonometry are used to measure IOP in children.

Corneal Measurements

- Corneal Diameter:
- Measurement: Corneal diameter in infants is approximately 9.5–10 mm [12].
- Techniques: Measured using slit-lamp examination or corneal topography.
- Corneal Thickness:
- Measurement: Central corneal thickness in children typically ranges from 500 to 540 microns (μm). Abnormal thickness can indicate glaucomatous changes or other conditions.
- Techniques: Measured using pachymetry or OCT.

Optic Nerve Head (ONH) Parameters

- Cup-to-Disc Ratio:
- Measurement: Increased ratio can suggest glaucomatous damage. Normal ratios are generally <0.4 [13].
- Techniques: Evaluated using fundus photography, OCT, or Heidelberg Retinal Tomography (HRT).
- Optic Nerve Head (ONH) Cupping:
- Measurement: The depth and size of the optic nerve cup. Increased cupping can indicate glaucoma.

Retinal Nerve Fiber Layer (RNFL) Thickness

- Measurement:
- Normal Range: Typically, 90–120 microns (μm). Thinning of the RNFL is associated with glaucomatous damage.
- Techniques: Assessed using Optical Coherence Tomography (OCT).Visual Field Testing
- Measurement:
- Testing Methods: Age-appropriate methods such as automated perimetry for older children or behavioral tests for younger children to assess visual field defects.
- Techniques: Automated visual field tests, preferential looking tests, or electrophysiological tests.

Corneal Hysteresis

- Measurement:
- Normal Range: Typically, 8–12 mmHg. Reduced corneal hysteresis can be indicative of glaucomatous damage.
- Techniques: Measured using an ocular response analyzer.

Anterior Segment Imaging

- Measurement:
- Techniques: Provides detailed images of the anterior segment, including the angle, cornea, and lens. Used to assess angle structures and detect abnormalities.
- Techniques: Includes AS-OCT and Scheimpflug imaging.

Developmental and Functional Assessments

- Visual Development:
- Milestones: Assessing visual function and development at various ages, as children with glaucoma may have developmental delays or visual impairments.
- Techniques: Evaluating developmental milestones related to visual processing and response.
- Functional Tests:
- Measurement: Evaluates the impact of glaucoma on visual function, including tasks such as reading or recognizing objects.

Genetic and Systemic Evaluations

- Genetic Testing:
- Measurement: Identifying genetic mutations associated with congenital glaucoma or other hereditary forms. Common genes include MYOC, CYP1B1, and LTBP2.
- Systemic Conditions:
- Monitoring: Evaluating the impact of systemic conditions (e.g., Sturge-Weber syndrome) on ocular health.

Tear Production

- Measurement:
- Tear Film Break-Up Time (TBUT): Assessing tear production and stability, which can be affected by glaucoma or its treatment.
- Normal Range: Typically, greater than 10 s.

Of Related Interest Greater axial elongation during childhood growth caused a significant shift of the cpRNFL peaks toward the fovea and increased IT thickness. Based on the plate hypothesis, the shift and compression of nerve fibers during growth may serve as a potential predictor of normal-tension glaucoma onset in the future.

Yamashita T, Terasaki H, Asaoka R, Yoshihara N, Kakiuchi N, Sakamoto T. Longitudinal changes in the position and thickness of the peak peripapillary retinal nerve fiber layer in school children. Graefes Arch Clin Exp Ophthalmol. 2025;263(7):1977–84. Epub 2025 Mar 25. https://doi.org/10.1007/s00417-025-06810-z. PMID:40133724.

In *Pediatric Retina Research*, several measurements and parameters are crucial for understanding, diagnosing, and managing retinal conditions in children.

Retinal Imaging and Structure

- Retinal Thickness:
- Measurement: Retinal thickness is assessed using Optical Coherence Tomography (OCT). Normal thickness varies by retinal layer and age, and instrument used.
- Techniques: OCT provides cross-sectional images of the retina, helping to identify abnormalities including retinal edema or thinning.
- Retinal Layer Evaluation:

- Measurement: Detailed evaluation of retinal layers (e.g., ganglion cell layer, inner plexiform layer). Changes in thickness or structure can indicate conditions such as retinal dystrophies or diabetic retinopathy.
- Fundus Photography:
- Measurement: Provides detailed images of the retina, useful for assessing conditions such as retinopathy of prematurity (ROP), retinal detachment, or congenital retinal anomalies.

Retinal Blood Flow and Vascularization

- Retinal Blood Flow:
- Documentation: Assessed using techniques such as fluorescein angiography or OCT angiography to evaluate the blood vessels in the retina.
- Techniques: Fluorescein angiography involves injecting a dye to visualize blood flow, while OCT angiography provides a noninvasive method to visualize retinal blood vessels.
- Vascularization:
- Important in conditions such as ROP, where abnormal retinal vascular growth can occur.

Visual Function

- Visual Acuity:
- Measurement: Assessed using age-appropriate tests (e.g., visual acuity charts for older children, preferential looking tests for younger ones). Normal visual acuity improves from around 20/400 at birth to 20/20–2025 by about age 7 years.
- Electrophysiological Testing:
- Measurement: Includes Electroretinography (ERG) to measure the electrical response of the retina to light stimuli. Useful for diagnosing retinal degenerative diseases.

Retinal Development

- Retinal Maturation:
- Measurement: The retina continues to mature throughout childhood, with changes in thickness, vascularization, and function. Monitoring these changes is important for assessing normal development and detecting abnormalities.

Retinal Detachment and Disorders

- Retinal Detachment:
- Measurement: Assessing the extent and location of retinal detachment using OCT, fundus photography, and ultrasound.
- Techniques: B-scan ultrasound can help visualize detachment in cases where fundus view is limited.
- Retinal Disorders:
- Measurement: Includes assessing for conditions such as retinal dystrophies, ROP, and macular holes. Techniques include OCT, fundus photography, and genetic testing for inherited disorders.

Ocular Biometry

- Axial Length:
- Measurement: The length of the eye from the front to the back, measured using ultrasonography or OCT. Normal axial length in children is typically 22–24 millimeters (mm), and significant deviations can indicate conditions such as myopia or hyperopia.
- Anterior Chamber Depth:
- Measurement: Measured using OCT or ultrasound. Important for assessing anterior segment conditions and planning for surgeries if needed.

In *Low Vision Rehabilitation Research*, numerical values, standards, and units are commonly used to measure visual function, level of visual impairment, and the effectiveness of vision rehabilitation interventions. Low vision rehabilitation research focuses on understanding, improving, and developing interventions and technologies for visually impaired or blind individuals to maximize their functional vision, maintain independence, and improve quality of life. Current research includes investigating the effectiveness of various assistive technologies such as head mounted displays (e.g., IrisVision, eSight), text-to-speech software or devices (e.g., OrCam, Meta glasses), navigation tools, advancements in retinal or cortical implants, and integration of artificial intelligence (AI). Other research avenues include tele-rehabilitation, gene therapies, the psychosocial and cognitive aspects of visual impairment, researching barriers to care, and investigating the causes and prevalence and demographics of visual impairment and blindness.

Visual Acuity (VA)

- Snellen Fraction: The most common unit of measurement for visual acuity.
  - Example: 20/20 (normal vision), 20/40 (visual impairment), 20/200 (considered legally blind if 20/200 is the best corrected acuity in the BETTER seeing eye).
- LogMAR: Another common measure of visual acuity used in research. It is a logarithmic scale, where 0.0 represents 20/20 vision, and higher values indicate worse acuity.
  - Example: LogMAR of 0.3 corresponds to 20/40 vision.

Visual Field (VF)

- Degrees of Visual Field: The extent of the visual field is measured in degrees. Normal visual field in one eye is a total of 150° horizontally and 130° vertically. There is a physiological overlap of the nasal portion of the visual field of each eye.
  - Central vision: 0–20°
  - Mid-peripheral: 20°–60°
  - Peripheral vision: 60° and beyond
- Goldmann Perimeter: Used to measure the extent of visual fields quantitatively, with values reported in isopters (lines representing the threshold of vision at different locations). Isopters can be brighter or dimmer and larger or smaller.

Isopters are notated by a Roman numeral, a number, and a lowercase letter (e.g., III4e, V4e). The higher the Roman numeral the larger the target is and therefore the easier it is to detect.
- Automated Perimetry: Reports the threshold sensitivity of the visual field in decibels (dB), where higher values indicate a higher sensitivity threshold.

Contrast Sensitivity (CS)
- Units: Contrast sensitivity is often measured in cycles per degree (cpd), assessing the ability to detect differences in luminance between an object and its background.
  - Normal CS: 2–4 cpd.
- Pelli-Robson Chart: A test for contrast sensitivity. The threshold is reported in log units.
- Vistech CS Testing: Also used in research, reporting values of contrast sensitivity at various spatial frequencies.

Reading Speed
- Words Per Minute (WPM): A standard measure to assess the speed of reading with low vision aids. This is a common functional outcome measure in low vision rehabilitation studies. The MNRead near card is a commonly near visual acuity test used in many research studies.
- Reading acuity: Measured using reading charts, often reported as the minimum angle of resolution (MAR), and can also be related to reading speed.

Low Vision Classification
- Visual Impairment Categories (based on WHO and legal definitions):
  - Mild Visual Impairment: 20/30 to 20/60.
  - Moderate Visual Impairment: 20/70 to 20/160.
  - Severe Visual Impairment: 20/200 to 20/400.
  - Blindness: 20/500 to 20/1000 (or worse).
  - Legally Blind: 20/200 or worse in the better-seeing eye, or visual field of less than 20 degrees.

Foveal Vision and Macular Function
- Foveal Sensitivity: A measure of the most sensitive central 1–2° of vision, often assessed with microperimetry.
- Macular Pigment Optical Density: A measure that helps assess macular health, often used in conditions like age-related macular degeneration.
- Fixation Stability: Measured in degrees or in terms of the number of saccades (eye movements) required to maintain fixation.

Quality of Life (QoL) and Functional Vision Assessment
- National Eye Institute Visual Function Questionnaire (NEI-VFQ-25): A standardized tool used to assess how visual impairment impacts daily living.
  - Scores range from 0 (worst) to 100 (best) for various functional categories.

- Visual Disability Rating Scale: Another tool for measuring the impact of low vision on daily activities.

Distance and Near Vision Performance
- Near Acuity: Measured in terms of Snellen equivalents or LogMAR at standard distances (e.g., 40 cm for near vision).
- Near Working Distance: The distance at which a patient performs common activities (e.g., reading, writing, using a computer).
- Distance Vision: Typically measured at 6 meters (20 feet) using the ETDRS chart (Early Treatment of Diabetic Retinopathy Study), Colenbrander Mixed Contrast chart, or Snellen.

Eye Movement and Fixation
- Saccadic Movements: Eye movements used to rapidly shift fixation from one object to another, typically quantified in degrees per second.
- Fixation Duration: Measured in milliseconds, with research often focusing on how fixation duration correlates with reading ability or reading speed and other visual tasks.

Luminance and Illumination Levels
- Lux: A unit of measurement for light intensity, commonly used to evaluate lighting conditions in low vision research.
  - Low vision individuals may require lighting conditions of 500–1000 lux for optimal function, compared to normal conditions of 300–500 lux.

Binocular Vision and Accommodation
- Inter-pupillary Distance (IPD): The distance between the centers of the pupils in each eye, often measured in millimeters (mm).
- Accommodation Range: The ability of the eye to change focus, typically measured in diopters (D).
- Vergences: The ability of the eyes to converge or diverge, measured in prism diopters (Δ).

Low Vision Aids and Devices
- Magnification Level: Often expressed as the magnification power, such as 2×, 4×, or 6× magnification.
- Field of View: The amount of visual field available when using devices like telescopes measured in degrees.
- Reading Rate with Aids: Words per minute (WPM) when using magnifiers or other assistive devices.

Statistical and Research Parameters
- Effect Size: A statistical measure used in low vision research to quantify the strength of the effect of interventions or treatments.
- Confidence Interval (CI): Often used in low vision research studies to indicate the reliability of results (e.g., 95% CI).

- P-values: Statistical significance often reported to determine the effectiveness of interventions or comparisons (typically <0.05).

Peripheral Vision

- Visual Field Loss: Measured in degrees of loss, often reporting "field defects" such as "right superior quadrant loss" or "nasal field loss."
- Central Versus Peripheral Vision: Research often distinguishes between central vision (0–20°) and peripheral vision (beyond 20–30°), as they affect various visual tasks differently.

Age-Related Changes

- Presbyopia: The age-related decline in near vision, usually occurring around the age of 40.
- Age-Related Macular Degeneration (AMD): Often assessed in terms of visual acuity (VA) and field loss, with specific categorization of stages (early, intermediate, late) [14, 15]

Of Related Interest Optogenetics involves introducing light-sensitive proteins into retinal cells allowing them to respond to light and restore visual function. This technique holds potential for patients with advanced photoreceptor loss.

Sahel JA, et al. Partial recovery of visual function in a blind patient after optogenetic therapy. Nat Med. 2021;27(7):1223–9. https://doi.org/10.1038/s41591-021-01351-4.

References

1. Enaholo ES, Musa MJ, Zeppieri M. Optical coherence tomography. In: StatPearls [Internet]. Treasure Island: StatPearls Publishing; 2025. Updated 2024 Oct 6. Available from: https://www.ncbi.nlm.nih.gov/books/NBK606122/.
2. Böhm EW, Pfeiffer N, Wagner FM, Gericke A. Methods to measure blood flow and vascular reactivity in the retina. Front Med (Lausanne). 2023;9:1069449. https://doi.org/10.3389/fmed.2022.1069449.
3. Tan B, Chua J, Wong D, Liu X, Ismail M, Schmetterer L. Techniques for imaging the choroid and choroidal blood flow in vivo. Exp Eye Res. 2024;247:110045. https://doi.org/10.1016/j.exer.2024.110045.
4. Motamed Shariati M, Khazaei S, Yaghoobi M. Choroidal vascularity index in health and systemic diseases: a systematic review. Int J Retina Vitreous. 2024;10:87. https://doi.org/10.1186/s40942-024-00607-8.
5. Puri S, Shaikh AG. Basic and translational neuro-ophthalmology of visually guided saccades: disorders of velocity. Expert Rev Ophthalmol. 2017;12(6):457–73. https://doi.org/10.1080/17469899.2017.1395695.
6. Lamb TD. Evolution of phototransduction, vertebrate photoreceptors and retina. Prog Retin Eye Res. 2013;36:52–119. https://doi.org/10.1016/j.preteyeres.2013.06.001.
7. Wu H, de Boer JF, Chen TC. Reproducibility of retinal nerve fiber layer thickness measurements using spectral domain optical coherence tomography. J Glaucoma. 2011;20(8):470–6. https://doi.org/10.1097/IJG.0b013e3181f3eb64.

8. Wolffsohn JS, Davies LN. Advances in anterior segment imaging. Curr Opin Ophthalmol. 2007;18(1):32–8. https://doi.org/10.1097/ICU.0b013e328011550d.
9. Hall JC. Visual evoked potentials: basic concepts and clinical applications. J Clin Neurophysiol. 2015;32(6):461–70.
10. Shields CL, Shields JA. Tumors of the eye. In: Yanoff M, Duker JS, editors. Ophthalmology. 3rd ed. Philadelphia: Elsevier; 2009. p. 1345–416.
11. Levine MR, Allen RC, editors. Manual of oculoplastic surgery. 5th ed. New York: Springer; 2018. Available from: https://link.springer.com/content/pdf/10.1007/978-3-319-74512-1.pdf
12. Freedman S. In: Becker B, Shaffer RN, editors. Diagnosis and therapy of the glaucomas. C.V. Mosby: St Louis; 1965.
13. Richardson KT. Optic cup symmetry in normal newborn infants. Invest Ophthalmol. 1968;7:137–47.
14. Massof RW, Goldstein JE, Deremeik JT, et al. Functional outcomes and quality of life in low vision rehabilitation. In: Jackson ML, Fletcher DC, Fontenot JL, editors. Vision rehabilitation for adults. San Francisco: American Academy of Ophthalmology; 2012. p. 102–18.
15. Yuan SM, Rafaelof M, Huang JD, Mehta MC. Head-mounted devices for low vision: a review. Int Ophthalmol Clin. 2025;65(1):53–8.

Chapter 14
Key Values of Therapeutic Lasers Used in Ophthalmology

- Excimer Laser (cornea):
  - Wavelength: 193 nm
  - Fluence: 100–300 mJ/cm^2 (millijoules per square centimeter)
  - Pulse Duration: 20–30 ns (nanoseconds)
  - Ablation Rate: 0.25–0.5 microns per pulse
  - Spot Size: 0.6 mm in diameter
- Femtosecond Laser (refractive, and cataract surgery):
  - Wavelength: 1053 nm
  - Pulse Duration: 200 fs (femtoseconds)
  - Spot Size: 1–2 microns
- YAG Laser (lens, posterior capsule opacification):
  - Wavelength: 1064 nm
  - Pulse Duration: 5–10 ns
  - Energy Output: 6–10 mJ per pulse
- Diode Laser (retina):
  - Wavelength: Range of 810 nm to 980 nm.
  - Power: Range is 50–300 mW.
  - Spot Size: Range of 50–200 microns.
- Argon Laser (retina):
  - Wavelength: 488 nm and 514 nm (blue-green light)
  - Power: Usually 50–1500 mW
  - Pulse Duration: Continuous wave or pulsed [1]

M. P. Kelly, *Normal Values in Vision Science*,
https://doi.org/10.1007/978-3-032-18207-4_14

It is important to note that ophthalmic device manufacturers may use different methods leading to variations in the numeric values their devices report as compared to competitor devices; the information provided here should not be used to adjust device settings or guide treatment decisions.

Reference

1. Zhang AY, Kumar D, Tripathy K. Laser principles in ophthalmology. In: StatPearls [Internet]. Treasure Island: StatPearls Publishing; 2023. [cited 2025 Aug 17]. Available from: https://www.ncbi.nlm.nih.gov/books/NBK582153/.

Chapter 15
Normative Databases in Ophthalmology and Vision Science

Normative databases in ophthalmology and vision science are collections of reference data derived from healthy individuals. These datasets serve as benchmarks for evaluating eye structure and visual function, playing a critical role in clinical decision-making. By comparing a patient's results to normative values, clinicians can detect early signs of ocular disease, often before symptoms emerge. This allows for timely diagnosis, monitoring, and treatment of conditions such as glaucoma, diabetic retinopathy, and age-related macular degeneration.

These databases include data stratified by demographics including age, gender, and ethnicity, accounting for natural variations across populations. In clinical settings, they support precise interpretation of test results, while in research, they enable the study of population trends, risk factors, and genetic influences on eye health. As they evolve, normative databases are expected to contribute to the development of more personalized and precision-based approaches to eye care.

Normative Databases for Optical Coherence Tomography (OCT)

Normative databases are especially vital in optical coherence tomography (OCT), a high-resolution, noninvasive imaging technology used to visualize cross-sectional details of the retina and optic nerve head. OCT normative databases provide standard measurements for:

- Retinal thickness
- Choroidal thickness
- Retinal nerve fiber layer (RNFL) thickness
- Optic nerve head parameters

M. P. Kelly, *Normal Values in Vision Science*,
https://doi.org/10.1007/978-3-032-18207-4_15

These values serve as essential references for identifying structural abnormalities in patients and are foundational for diagnosing and tracking conditions such as glaucoma, macular degeneration, diabetic retinopathy, and inherited retinal diseases.

Population Size and Diversity
To generate reliable normative data, studies typically include at least 200–300 healthy eyes, though the required sample size depends on factors such as:

- Statistical power
- Population heterogeneity (age, gender, ethnicity)
- Device specifications

The demographic diversity of the sample is critical, as key parameters—such as retinal thickness and RNFL thickness—can vary significantly across ethnic and age groups.

Device and Measurement Variability
Normative values can differ across OCT platforms (e.g., spectral-domain vs. time-domain OCT) due to variations in:

- Imaging technology
- Scan protocols
- Segmentation algorithms

Therefore, care must be taken when comparing patient data acquired from different devices or when monitoring progression over time using multiple systems.

Clinical and Research Utility
A robust normative database allows clinicians to:

- Accurately distinguish between normal anatomical variation and disease
- Monitor changes over time with confidence
- Tailor interpretations for individual patients based on demographic context

For researchers, these databases facilitate:

- Epidemiological studies
- Development of diagnostic algorithms
- Insights into disease pathophysiology

As imaging technologies and AI integration advance, normative databases will continue to evolve, enhancing diagnostic accuracy and supporting precision medicine in ophthalmology.

Of Related Interest Personalized Medicine in the Making: Philosophical Perspectives from Biology to Healthcare brings together top scholars on the debated concept of personalized medicine and addresses the topic from a multidisciplinary point of view. https://doi.org/10.1007/978-3-030-74804-3

Challenges in Establishing Pediatric Normative Data for OCT and OCT-A

Creating robust normative databases for optical coherence tomography (OCT) and OCT-angiography (OCTA) in infants and children is challenging. These imaging techniques are sensitive and provide detailed data on retinal and vascular structures, but their application across a developing age group introduces several scientific, technical, and logistical hurdles. Additionally, these measurements are influenced by age, refraction, gender, and ethnicity.

1. Ongoing Ocular Development
   - The retina, fovea, choroid, optic nerve head, and vasculature all undergo structural and functional maturation from birth into adolescence.
   - Normative values vary not only by age, but also by:
     - Axial length
     - Refraction
     - Retinal layer thickness
     - Vascular density
   - Unlike adults, *normal* values in children are dynamic, and any database must be age-stratified and growth-adjusted.
2. Limited Cooperation and Motion Artifacts
   - Young children, especially infants and toddlers, cannot consistently fixate or remain still.
   - This leads to:
     - Motion artifacts
     - Segmentation errors
     - Lower image quality
   - Handheld OCT devices have improved accessibility, but they still lack the quantitative metrics/analytics and reproducibility of table-mounted devices.
3. Small Sample Sizes
   - Ethical and logistical issues limit large-scale recruitment.
   - The use of sedation (if needed) raises ethical concerns, and parental consent must be obtained.
   - Many studies are single-center, limiting diversity in ethnicity, geography, and socioeconomic status.
4. Lack of Standardization Across Devices and Algorithms
   - Different OCT/OCTA platforms use different software, segmentation protocols, and layer definitions.
   - Pediatric eyes have different morphologies than adult eyes, and many automated algorithms are not validated for children.

- Manual correction is time-consuming and introduces interobserver variability.

5. Axial Length and Refractive Error Correction

- Axial length changes significantly with age, especially in the first few years.
- OCT image magnification is affected by axial length, which can distort thickness and vascular density measurements.
- Pediatric normative databases need to incorporate axial length scaling or risk inaccurate comparisons.

6. Vascular Development and Variability in OCT-A

- Retinal vascular development continues postnatally (especially in preterm infants), influencing vessel density, FAZ (foveal avascular zone), and perfusion indices.
- OCTA is also susceptible to:
  - Motion
  - Projection artifacts
  - Incorrect segmentation of capillary plexuses
- Robust norms must therefore be age-specific and adjusted for the stage of retinal vascular maturation.

Foveal Development and FAZ on OCT-A

- In neonates and infants, the foveal avascular zone (FAZ) may be absent or ill defined.
- The FAZ expands and the surrounding capillary plexus matures over time, affecting interpretation of OCT-A data. The reorganization of the foveal zone during childhood may explain the difference in macular thickness with age [1–4].

References

1. Maldonado RS, Toth CA. Optical coherence tomography in retinopathy of prematurity: looking beyond the vessels. Clin Perinatol. 2013;40(2):271–96. https://doi.org/10.1016/j.clp.2013.02.007.
2. Lee H, Proudlock FA, Gottlob I. Is handheld optical coherence tomography reliable in infants and young children with and without nystagmus? Invest Ophthalmol Vis Sci. 2013;54(13):8152–9. https://doi.org/10.1167/iovs.13-13230.
3. Turk A, Ceylan OM, Arici C, Keskin S, Erdurman C, Durukan AH, Altintaş AG. Macular and retinal nerve fiber layer thickness in healthy children measured with spectral domain optical coherence tomography. J Pediatr Ophthalmol Strabismus. 2012;49(5):304–11. https://doi.org/10.3928/01913913-20120822-02. PMID: 22928603
4. Doblhoff-Dier V, Schuller SS, Neumann M, Salas M, Kraker H, Velikay-Parel M, Kroh ME, Krug AW, Brandstetter C, Prokesch V, Scholl-Bürgi S, Eder HG, Scharinger A, Benesch T, Ertl C, Glatz W, Siller B, Kirchmair R, Kieselbach G. Vascular development of the human fovea assessed by optical coherence tomography angiography. JAMA Ophthalmol. 2020;138(9):944–51. https://doi.org/10.1001/jamaophthalmol.2020.2277. PMID: 32609329

Chapter 16
Key Values in Current Imaging and Testing Technology

Ophthalmic Ultrasound is a noninvasive imaging technique that uses high-frequency sound waves to visualize structures within and around the eye. It is especially valuable when the view of the retina and other internal structures is blocked by media opacities, such as dense cataracts, vitreous hemorrhage, or corneal scarring.

A-Scan Biometry (A-scan is Amplitude scan) Primarily used to measure the axial length of the eye, often for calculating intraocular lens (IOL) power before cataract surgery.

Axial Length (AL)
- Normal range: 22.0–24.5 mm.
- Myopia: >24.5 mm.
- Hyperopia: <22.0 mm.

Anterior Chamber Depth (ACD)
- Normal range: 3.0–3.5 mm.

Lens Thickness (LT)
- Normal range: 4.0–5.0 mm.

Speed of Sound for Eye Components:
- Cornea: 1640 m/s.
- Aqueous: 1532 m/s.
- Lens: 1641–1648 m/s.
- Vitreous: 1532 m/s.

B-Scan Imaging (B-scan is Brightness Scan) Produces two-dimensional, cross-sectional images of the eye and orbit, helping diagnose conditions including retinal detachment, tumors, vitreous hemorrhage, and optic nerve abnormalities.

Standard Frequencies Used:
- 10 MHz: General-purpose imaging
- 20 MHz: Higher resolution but less penetration (used for anterior segment)

M. P. Kelly, *Normal Values in Vision Science*,
https://doi.org/10.1007/978-3-032-18207-4_16

Common Pathologies Visualized:
- Retinal Detachment: Highly reflective echogenic line separating from the choroid.
- Choroidal Detachment: Dome-shaped echogenicity with smooth contours.
- Vitreous Hemorrhage: Moderate echogenicity, often mobile.

Probe Placement:
- Transverse Scans: Horizontal imaging of the posterior pole.
- Longitudinal Scans: Vertical sections of the globe and retina.

Gain Settings:
- Usually adjusted between 60 and 80 dB for better differentiation of structures.

Other Key Measurements in Ophthalmic Ultrasound

Optic Nerve Sheath Diameter (ONSD):
- Normal range: <5.0 mm (measured 3 mm behind the globe).
- Enlarged in cases of increased intracranial pressure.

IOL Power Calculation:
- Uses axial length and keratometry values with formulas like SRK/T, Holladay, or Haigis.

A-Scan Biometry Details

1. Posterior Chamber Depth (PCD):
    - Normal range: 10–11 mm.
2. Speed of Sound Assumptions for IOL Calculations:
    - Average assumed speed: 1555 m/s.
    - Critical for accurate lens power determination, as deviations affect biometry precision.
3. Standard Axial Length Variability Impact:
    - 1 mm axial length error translates to ~3 diopters of refractive error in an intraocular lens (IOL) calculation.

B-Scan Imaging: Detailed Pathology Parameters

1. Retinal Detachment:
    - High reflectivity (strong echoes) on real-time dynamic imaging.
    - Moves less than vitreous structures during eye motion.

2. Vitreous Hemorrhage:
   - Mobile, low- to moderate-echogenic particles.
   - Increased gain enhances visibility.
3. Choroidal Detachment:
   - Smooth, dome-shaped echoes, often bilobed.
   - Seen at low reflectivity compared to retinal detachment.
4. Intraocular Tumors:
   - Typically high internal reflectivity (depends on the tumor type; Uveal melanoma has low internal reflectivity, for example).
   - Dome-shaped or irregular mass adherent to the sclera.
5. Posterior Vitreous Detachment (PVD):
   - Highly reflective, mobile linear echoes.

Anterior Segment Ultrasound Biomicroscopy (UBM) is a high-frequency ultrasound imaging technique (typically 35–50 MHz) used to obtain detailed, high-resolution images of the anterior segment of the eye. Unlike standard B-scan ultrasound, which focuses on posterior structures, UBM allows clinicians to visualize microscopic anatomy of the front of the eye including the cornea, iris, ciliary body, anterior chamber angle, and lens zonules.

1. Frequency Range for UBM Probes:
   - 35–50 MHz (high-frequency imaging for detailed anterior segment structures)
2. Common Measurements in UBM:
   - Angle Opening Distance (AOD):
   - Measured at 500 μm from the scleral spur.
   - Normal: >0.3 mm.
   - Trabecular-Iris Angle (TIA):
   - Normal: >25°.
   - Ciliary Body Thickness (CBT):
   - Normal: 0.8–1.2 mm.
3. Anterior Chamber Angle (ACA):
   - Narrow ACA: <20°.
   - Wide ACA: >30°.

Orbital Ultrasound (B-Scan) is a diagnostic imaging technique that uses high-frequency sound waves to generate two-dimensional, cross-sectional images of the globe and orbit.

1. Optic Nerve Sheath Diameter (ONSD):
    - <5 mm: Normal
    - >5.5 mm: Suggestive of raised intracranial pressure
2. Muscle Thickness (EOM Evaluation):
    - Superior rectus muscle: 4–6 mm.
    - Inferior rectus muscle: 4–6 mm.
    - Increased thickness seen in Graves' orbitopathy or orbital pseudotumor.
3. Lesions:
    - Cystic Lesions: Low internal reflectivity, well-demarcated.
    - Solid Lesions: Higher reflectivity, often irregular.

Specialized Diagnostic Values

1. Vitreous Opacities:
    - Echogenicity varies; better detected with dynamic eye movement.
2. Ocular Trauma:
    - Intraocular Foreign Body: Highly echogenic, often with posterior shadowing.
    - Hyphema/Choroidal Hemorrhage: Moderate to high reflectivity, depending on clot age.
3. Measurement of Axial Length in Trauma Cases:
    - Axial length discrepancy: Compare injured to healthy eye.
    - Shortened axial length may indicate globe rupture [1, 2].

Optical Coherence Tomography (OCT) is a noninvasive imaging technology that uses low-coherence light to capture high-resolution, cross-sectional images of the eye's internal structures, particularly the retina, macula, optic nerve head, and anterior segment.

Retinal Layers and Thicknesses

1. Central Macular Thickness (CMT):
    - Normal range: 250–300 μm (varies slightly with age and device used).
    - Increased in macular edema (e.g., diabetic macular edema or retinal vein occlusion).
    - Decreased in atrophic conditions like macular degeneration or advanced glaucoma.

2. Retinal Nerve Fiber Layer (RNFL) Thickness (Glaucoma):
    - Normal average: ~90–110 μm (measured around the optic nerve head).
    - <80 μm: Suggestive of glaucoma progression.
    - Sector-specific values: Superior and inferior quadrants are typically thicker than nasal or temporal quadrants.
3. Ganglion Cell Complex (GCC) Thickness (Glaucoma/Neuropathy):
    - Normal average: varies, roughly 80–110 μm (differs due to age, sex, race, device used, segmentation applied, etc.)
    - Decreased in optic neuropathy and early glaucoma.

Retinal Zones in Disease Monitoring

1. Ellipsoid Zone (EZ):
    - Normal: Continuous, hyper-reflective band.
    - Disruption: Marker for photoreceptor damage (e.g., AMD, RP).
2. Subfoveal Choroidal Thickness (Choroidopathies):
    - Normal: ~200–300 μm in healthy adults.
    - Increased in conditions like central serous chorioretinopathy (CSC).
    - Decreased in high myopia or atrophic conditions.

OCT Angiographic and Morphometric Features

1. Macular Hole (Full-Thickness):
    - Small: <250 μm.
    - Medium: 250–400 μm.
    - Large: >400 μm.
2. Epiretinal Membrane (ERM):
    - Thickness varies; causes retinal distortion and irregular reflectivity of inner retinal layers.
3. Drusen (AMD):
    - Height and volume tracked longitudinally for progression.
    - Large drusen: >125 μm in diameter (Small: ≤63, Medium: >63 but ≤125).

Optical Coherence Tomography Angiography (OCTA) is a noninvasive imaging technique that visualizes blood flow in the retina and choroid without the need for dye injection. It builds on standard OCT technology by capturing motion contrast from red blood cells as they move through vessels, producing high-resolution 3D images of the microvasculature.

Vascular Metrics

1. Superficial Vascular Density (SVD):
    - Normal macular SVD: 40–55% (varies by device and age).
    - Reduced in ischemic diseases (e.g., diabetic retinopathy, retinal vein occlusion).
2. Foveal Avascular Zone (FAZ):
    - Normal area: 0.25–0.5 mm^2 (measured in the superficial capillary plexus).
    - Enlarged FAZ in ischemic conditions (e.g., diabetic retinopathy).
3. Vessel Density (VD):
    - Measured in superficial and deep retinal capillary plexuses.
    - Reduced VD seen in glaucoma and retinal vascular diseases.
4. Choriocapillaris Flow Void:
    - Evaluates hypoperfusion or ischemia.
    - Abnormal in conditions like AMD or uveitis.

Disease-Specific OCTA Metrics

1. Neovascularization (NV):
    - Measured as an increase in flow signal area (e.g., choroidal neovascularization in AMD).
2. Diabetic Retinopathy:
    - Capillary Non-Perfusion Areas: Quantified in mm^2.
    - Microaneurysms: Detected as small flow signal spots in vascular plexuses.
3. Glaucoma:
    - Peripapillary Vessel Density (PVD):
    - Normal: ~50–60%.
    - Decreased in glaucomatous optic neuropathy.

OCT Imaging Parameters

1. Axial Resolution:
   - Typical resolution: ~5–7 μm (Spectral-Domain OCT).
   - Enhanced resolution: ~2–3 μm (Swept-Source OCT).
2. Scan Depth:
   - Standard OCT: ~2–3 mm.
   - Swept-Source OCT: ~6–7 mm (ideal for choroidal imaging).
3. Scan Speed:
   - Spectral-Domain OCT: ~30,000–70,000 A-scans/second.
   - Swept-Source OCT: ~100,000–200,000 A-scans/second [3].

Key numbers and parameters relevant to Ophthalmic Electrophysiology, including electroretinogram (ERG), electro-oculogram (EOG), and visual evoked potentials (VEP). These measurements are essential for diagnosing and monitoring retinal and visual pathway disorders.

1. *Electroretinogram (ERG).*

   (a) Full-Field ERG (ISCEV Standard Parameters).

   1. Scotopic (Dark-Adapted) Responses:
      - Rod Response (Low-Intensity Stimulus):
        - Amplitude: 100–300 μV.
        - Implicit time: ~100 ms.
      - Maximal Combined Response (Bright Flash):
        - a-wave: Amplitude: 100–200 μV, Time to peak: 10–15 ms,
        - b-wave: Amplitude: 200–600 μV, Time to peak: 30–50 ms,
   2. Photopic (Light-Adapted) Responses:
      - Cone Response (Flicker ERG):
        - Amplitude: 10–50 μV.
        - Implicit time: 25–30 ms (30 Hz flicker).
      - Single Flash Cone Response:
        - a-wave: Amplitude: 10–20 μV, Time to peak: 10–15 ms,
        - b-wave: Amplitude: 50–100 μV, Time to peak: 25–35 ms.
   3. Oscillatory Potentials:
      - Amplitude: 10–40 μV (sum of waves).
      - Delays or reductions suggest ischemic conditions (e.g., diabetic retinopathy).

(b) *Multifocal ERG (mfERG).*

1. Amplitude (First-Order Kernel):

   - Central retina: ~40–50 nV/deg^2.
   - Peripheral retina: ~10–20 nV/deg^2.

2. Implicit Time (First-Order Kernel):

   - Normal: 30–35 ms (varies with eccentricity).

2. *Electro-Oculogram (EOG).*

(a) Arden Ratio (Light/Dark Ratio):

- Normal range: >1.8.
- Subnormal range: 1.65–1.8.
- Abnormal range: <1.65.

(b) Light Peak Latency:

- Normal: ~8–12 minutes after light onset4.

(c) Baseline Dark Voltage:

- Normal: 200–500 μV.

3. Visual Evoked Potentials (VEP).

(a) Pattern VEP (ISCEV Standard Parameters).

1. P100 Latency (Checkerboard Pattern Reversal):

   - Normal: 90–120 ms (depends on age and check size).
   - Delayed in optic neuropathies (e.g., multiple sclerosis).

2. P100 Amplitude:

   - Normal: 5–10 μV (peak-to-peak).
   - Reduced in conditions like amblyopia or optic nerve damage.

3. Check Sizes:

   - Small Checks (6–12 minutes of arc): Higher cortical activity, longer latency.
   - Large Checks (60 minutes of arc): Shorter latency but reduced amplitude.

(b) Flash VEP.

1. P2 Latency:

   - Normal: ~100–125 ms.
   - Used when pattern VEP is unrecordable (e.g., severe media opacity).

2. Amplitude:

   - Normal: ~3–10 μV [4, 5].

Dark Adaptation evaluates how well the eye adjusts from bright to dim lighting conditions—a process largely dependent on rod photoreceptor function in the retina. It is an important functional test used to detect early retinal dysfunction, especially in diseases affecting the retinal pigment epithelium (RPE) and photoreceptors (see also a later section in this book on same subject).

1. Rod Threshold Recovery (10° Off-Fovea):

   - Normal: ~10–20 minutes to recover to baseline sensitivity.

Photopic Negative Response (PhNR):
- Amplitude: 10–30 μV below baseline.
- Reduced in inner retinal diseases like glaucoma [6].

Retinal Response Latencies:
- Rod-driven responses: ~20–30 ms slower than cone-driven responses due to slower kinetics [7].

These values represent typical reference ranges and may vary based on equipment and patient factors (e.g., age, refractive error). In particular, Dawson-Trick-Litzkow (DTL) electrodes produce larger ERG amplitudes than contact lens electrodes (Burian-Allen or Jet).

Key numbers and metrics relevant to *Ophthalmic Visual Field Testing*, primarily using automated perimetry (e.g., Humphrey Field Analyzer [HFA]) and Goldmann perimetry:

1. General Visual Field Dimensions.

   (a) Normal Visual Field Extent:

      - Superior: ~60°.
      - Inferior: ~75°.
      - Nasal: ~60°.
      - Temporal: ~100–110°.

2. Key Parameters in Automated Perimetry.

   (a) Threshold Values.

      1. Sensitivity Range (Normal Vision):

         - Central visual field: 26–38 dB.
         - Peripheral visual field: Decreases to 10–20 dB.
         - Maximum achievable sensitivity: 40 dB (depends on device calibration).

      2. Threshold Measurement Units:

         - Decibels (dB): Logarithmic scale of sensitivity (higher = better sensitivity).

(b) Pattern Deviation (PD).

- Highlights localized defects by adjusting for generalized depression (e.g., cataract).
- Normal Range: Values near 0 dB.

(c) Mean Deviation (MD) Hoddap-Anderson-Parrish criteria:

- Indicates overall deviation from normal sensitivity.
- Normal: Close to 0 dB.
- Mild Visual Field Loss: −2 to −6 dB.
- Moderate Loss: −6 to −12 dB.
- Severe Loss: <−12 dB.

(d) Visual Field Index (VFI):

- Percentage representing overall function of the visual field.
- 100%: Normal field
- <50%: Significant damage (e.g., late-stage glaucoma)

(e) Fixation Losses (Reliability):

- <20% is acceptable in reliable tests.

(f) False Positives/Negatives:

- False Positives (Trigger-Happy): Should be <15%.
- False Negatives (Missed Stimuli): Should be <20% [8].

3. *Key Parameters for Goldmann Perimetry*. Goldmann Visual Field (GVF) testing is a manual kinetic perimetry method still valued in certain clinical settings, particularly for patients with low vision, neurologic disease, or atypical field defects. It provides both qualitative and quantitative data.

(a) Stimulus Intensities:

- Range: Goldmann I (dim) to V (bright).
- Used for assessing large scotomas or peripheral field loss.

(b) Normal Kinetic Field Boundaries:

- Similar to static testing: Temporal extends up to 110°; nasal 60°.

4. Common Visual Field Defect Patterns.

(a) Glaucoma:

- Early Defects: Paracentral scotomas, nasal step.
- Advanced: Arcuate scotomas, generalized depression, or tunnel vision.

(b) Neurological Defects:

- Bitemporal hemianopia (chiasmal compression).
- Homonymous hemianopia (post-chiasmal lesions).

(c) Retinal Conditions:

- Central scotoma (macular disease).
- Ring scotoma (retinitis pigmentosa).

5. Specialized Tests and Numbers.

(a) Central 10-2 Visual Fields.

- Used for macular diseases or advanced glaucoma.
- Normal sensitivity: ~30–35 dB centrally.
- Reduced in conditions like AMD or advanced optic neuropathy.

(b) 24-2 Versus 30-2 Testing

- 24-2: Tests central 24° with 54 points. Common for glaucoma monitoring.
- 30-2: Tests central 30° with 76 points.

(c) Stimulus Size (Goldmann III or V):

- Goldmann III: Default size for standard perimetry.
- Larger stimuli (e.g., V) used for patients with poor vision or extensive field loss.

(d) Scotoma Size Definitions:

- Absolute Scotoma: No sensitivity (0 dB).
- Relative Scotoma: Sensitivity is reduced compared to expected norms.

Goldmann Visual Field Numbers At-A-Glance:

- Test Radius: 90° (from fixation to periphery).
- Stimulus Size (Roman numerals I–V):
  - Size I: 0.25 mm^2.
  - Size II: 1.0 mm^2.
  - Size III: 4.0 mm^2 (standard in automated perimetry, for comparison).
  - Size IV: 16.0 mm^2.
  - Size V: 64.0 mm^2 (used in low vision or tunnel vision cases).
- Intensity Levels (Arabic numbers 1–4 with a–e steps):
  - 1a (dim) to 4e (brightest)
  - Each step = 0.5 log unit change (about 5 dB).
  - Example: III4e means:
    - Size III (4 mm^2), Intensity 4e (maximum brightness).

Key Isopters

- III4e: Commonly used reference isopter.
  - Extends to ~60° temporally, ~50° inferiorly, ~50° superiorly, and ~ 60° nasally in normal vision.
- I4e: Smaller, dimmer target—used to detect early scotomas.
- V4e: Large, bright stimulus—used in low vision or advanced disease.

Normal Visual Field Extent (Approximate with III4e Stimulus)

Meridian	Degrees from fixation
Temporal	~90–100°
Nasal	~60°
Superior	~60°
Inferior	~70°

Scotoma Definitions

- Central scotoma: Within 5–10° of fixation.
- Paracentral scotoma: 10–30° from fixation.
- Peripheral constriction: Visual field limited to <20° radius → significant functional impairment (e.g., legal blindness) [9].

Of Related Interest Goldmann Visual Field (GVF) testing has been utilized in FDA-approved gene therapy trials for inherited retinal diseases, particularly in the evaluation of voretigene neparvovec-rzyl (Luxturna) for RPE65-mediated retinal dystrophy. In the pivotal Phase 3 clinical trial for Luxturna, GVF testing was employed to assess changes in visual field area as a secondary outcome measure. Specifically, the study used III4e and V4e stimuli to evaluate kinetic visual fields. It is fascinating that the Goldmann perimeter was introduced into clinical ophthalmology in *1945* by Hans Goldmann at the University of Bern, Switzerland, and quickly became the standard for manual kinetic perimetry, and still today is relied upon, in this instance for evaluating gene therapy trials in 2025, 80 years later.

Russell S, Bennett J, Wellman JA, et al. Efficacy and safety of voretigene neparvovec (AAV2-hRPE65v2) in patients with RPE65-mediated inherited retinal dystrophy: a randomised, controlled, open-label, phase 3 trial. Lancet. 2017;390(10097):849–60. https://doi.org/10.1016/S0140-6736(17)31868-8.

Microperimetry is a diagnostic tool used in ophthalmology to assess the functional vision of the retina, particularly in patients with retinal diseases such as age-related macular degeneration, diabetic retinopathy, and other conditions affecting visual function.

Key Values and Metrics

1. Threshold Sensitivity:
   - Measured in decibels (dB), this indicates the light intensity level at which a patient can detect a stimulus. Normal sensitivity typically ranges from 20 dB (poor) to 0 dB (excellent).
2. Visual Field Area:
   - The area of the visual field being tested, usually focusing on the macular region, which is critical for central vision.
3. Fixation Stability:
   - Measures the ability of the patient to maintain steady fixation on a target. This is crucial for interpreting sensitivity values. Fixation stability is often quantified as a percentage of time the patient maintained fixation within a certain radius of the target.
4. Sensitivity Maps:
   - Graphical representations that show the spatial distribution of retinal sensitivity. These maps can help identify localized areas of vision loss.
5. Mean Sensitivity:
   - The average sensitivity across all tested points in the visual field. This provides a general overview of retinal function.
6. Pointwise Sensitivity:
   - Sensitivity measured at specific points in the visual field, allowing for detailed assessment of localized areas.
7. Reproducibility:
   - The reliability of microperimetry results can be assessed through repeated testing, which shows how consistent the measurements are over time.

Important Considerations

- Age Norms: Normal sensitivity values can vary by age, with older patients often showing reduced sensitivity.
- Disease Impact: Different retinal diseases will have characteristic patterns of sensitivity loss, which can be compared against normative data.
- Testing Conditions: Ambient lighting, pupil size, and the patient's state on the day of testing can all influence microperimetry results.

Clinical Applications

- Monitoring Disease Progression: Microperimetry is often used to track changes in retinal sensitivity over time, helping to assess the progression of retinal diseases.
- Treatment Efficacy: It can be used to evaluate the effectiveness of treatments such as anti-VEGF injections in conditions like wet age-related macular degeneration.
- Surgical Planning: Microperimetry can assist in planning surgical interventions by providing detailed maps of functional vision.

Technologies and Devices

- MP-1: One of the commonly used microperimetry devices.
- MAIA: Another advanced device used for microperimetry that also provides additional features such as retinal imaging [10].

Contact Specular Microscopy provides detailed analysis of the endothelial cell layer of the human cornea. It is primarily used to evaluate corneal health, especially the integrity of the endothelium, which is vital for maintaining corneal transparency.

1. Endothelial Cell Density (ECD):
    - Normal range: 2000–3000 cells/mm^2 in adults.
    - Decline with age: ECD decreases by about 0.5% per year after childhood.
    - Threshold for concern: Values below 1000 cells/mm^2 may indicate significant endothelial dysfunction.
2. Cell Size (Polymegathism):
    - Coefficient of variation (CV): A measure of variability in cell size.
    - Normal value: <30%.
    - Higher values: Indicate polymegathism, often due to stress or damage (e.g., from contact lens wear or surgery).
3. Cell Shape (Pleomorphism):
    - Hexagonality: Percentage of cells with a hexagonal shape.
    - Normal value: ≥50%.
    - Lower values: Suggest pleomorphism, often linked to aging or corneal stress.
4. Central Corneal Thickness (CCT):
    - Often measured alongside endothelial assessment.
    - Normal range: 520–560 μm.
    - Thinner corneas: May indicate keratoconus or endothelial dysfunction.
    - Thicker corneas: May suggest corneal edema or inflammation.

5. Endothelial Guttae:

   - Presence of guttae (focal excrescences) can be a sign of Fuchs' endothelial dystrophy.
   - Evaluation includes noting their size, density, and coverage area.

These values help in diagnosing conditions like corneal endothelial dystrophies, evaluating pre- and post-operative health (e.g., cataract or keratoplasty surgeries), and monitoring corneal stress due to contact lens wear or trauma [11].

Dark Adaptation Testing is a valuable diagnostic tool in ophthalmology used to assess the ability of the retina, particularly the rod photoreceptors, to adjust to low-light conditions. Here are some key numbers and aspects related to dark adaptation testing in humans:

1. Duration of Testing: Dark adaptation testing typically lasts anywhere from 5 to 30 minutes, depending on the specific protocol. The time required for complete adaptation can vary among individuals.
2. Threshold Measurements: During dark adaptation tests, the sensitivity of the visual system is measured in terms of threshold light intensity. Normal thresholds for dark-adapted vision typically range from 0.1 to 1.0 photopic units (in terms of luminance), which corresponds to a sensitivity of approximately 20,000 to 50,000 times lower light intensity than what is required for photopic (daytime) vision.
3. Time Course of Adaptation: The dark adaptation process can be broken down into phases:

   - Cone Adaptation Phase: Occurs within the first 5–10 minutes in which the cone photoreceptors adapt to the dark.
   - Rod Adaptation Phase: Takes longer, with full rod adaptation usually occurring around 20 to 30 minutes. The rod photoreceptors are primarily responsible for vision in low-light conditions.

4. Sensitivity Improvement: Sensitivity to light can improve significantly during dark adaptation. After about 30 minutes in the dark, individuals may experience an increase in sensitivity by as much as 4 to 5 log units (10,000 to 100,000 times), compared to their initial sensitivity.
5. Clinical Significance: Dark adaptation testing can be used to detect various retinal disorders, including the following:

   - Retinitis pigmentosa.
   - Usher syndrome.
   - Vitamin A deficiency.
   - Diabetic retinopathy.

   Other diseases affecting night vision

6. Measurement Techniques: Various methods can be employed for dark adaptation testing, including the following:

- Static Threshold Testing: Measuring the light threshold after a set time in the dark.
- Kinetic Perimetry: Assessing the change in visual field sensitivity over time.

7. Age-Related Changes: Research indicates that dark adaptation may become slower with age, with older adults showing prolonged adaptation times compared to younger individuals [6, 7].

Key measurements and values associated with *Retinal Fundus Photography*:

1. Field of View (FOV)
   - Standard Field of View: single image up to 50°.
   - Wide Field of View: 60° to 100° depicting the posterior pole and including in a single image the areas posterior to the vortex vein ampulla in all four quadrants.
   - Ultra-Wide Field of View: 200° to 210° + in a single image including the posterior pole and out to areas anterior to the vortex vein ampulla in all four quadrants.
   - Montaging multiple images to create a wide field or ultrawide field composite image using standard or wide field imaging devices is indeed commonplace.
2. Resolution
   - Image Resolution: The resolution of a fundus image is typically between 1500 × 1500 pixels to 3000 × 3000 pixels, depending on the camera system.
   - Image Size: The size of a fundus image can range from 2 MB to over 10 MB depending on the camera's settings, such as resolution and color depth.
3. Color Depth
   - 8-bit or 16-bit color depth.
4. Light Intensity
   - Illumination: Retinal fundus cameras typically use a flash or LED light source with an intensity range of 100 to 500 lux. The brightness level needs to be adjusted to avoid retinal damage and to obtain clear images.
5. Pupil Size and Dilation
   - Undilated Pupils: 2–4 mm in diameter and requires a non-mydriatic retinal fundus camera; larger pupil equaling better quality image.
   - Dilated Pupils: After pharmacologic dilation, pupil size can range from 6 mm to 9 mm or more, depending on the drug used and the patient's individual reaction to the drug. Dilation facilitates successful capture of the peripheral retina.
6. Exposure Time
   - The shutter speed of the camera is 1/1000 to 1/250 of a second.

7. Optical Parameters

   - Working Distance: This can range from 10 mm to 50 mm between the eye and the camera's lens depending on the type of device used.
   - Magnification: Magnification factors can vary, often in the range of 1.0 to 2.5×.

8. Camera Systems and Type

   - Digital Versus Film-Based: Modern systems are primarily digital, offering advantages like high image quality, immediate analysis, and digital storage. Older systems used film, but digital has become the standard.
   - Camera Types: These may be non-mydriatic for undilated pupils or mydriatic, requiring pupil dilation.

9. Retinal Imaging Software

   - The software used for analyzing the fundus images may include specific features for image enhancement, retinal layer segmentation, and disease detection algorithms.

10. Color and Contrast

    - Fundus Imaging Colors: Fundus images are usually captured in RGB color space, and images are often presented in:

      – Color (RGB) for standard viewing.
      – Red-Free (removes red light to highlight retinal blood vessels).
      – Blue/Green for specific areas of interest (e.g., macular region or retinal layers).

    - Contrast Sensitivity: 10:1 contrast ratio.

11. Retinal Zones

    - Macula: The central area of the retina, responsible for detailed central vision, approximately 3 mm in diameter.
    - Optic Disc: The area where the optic nerve exits the retina, with a typical diameter of 1.5 mm.
    - Fovea: Located at the center of the macula, the fovea is around 0.35 mm in diameter [12].

Fundus Autofluorescence (FAF) is a noninvasive retinal imaging technique that captures the natural fluorescence of lipofuscin and other fluorophores within the retinal pigment epithelium (RPE). It provides valuable insights into the metabolic function and integrity of the RPE, helping in the diagnosis and monitoring of various retinal disorders.

FAF imaging involves exciting these fluorophores with specific wavelengths of light, most commonly blue at ~488 nm or, in some systems, green at 532–580. When excited, these compounds—particularly lipofuscin—emit autofluorescence that is detected in the 500–700 nm range, with peak emission around 600–630 nm.

The emitted light is captured using a confocal scanning laser ophthalmoscope (cSLO) or a fundus camera equipped for autofluorescence imaging.

FAF images reveal:

- Increased autofluorescence, often indicating lipofuscin accumulation or RPE stress.
- Decreased autofluorescence, suggesting RPE atrophy, cell loss, or hypopigmentation.

FAF is widely used in evaluating conditions such as:

- Age-related macular degeneration, including geographic atrophy.
- Stargardt's disease and other retinal dystrophies.
- Central serous chorioretinopathy (CSCR).
- Optic nerve drusen.
- Astrocytic hamartoma [13].

Fluorescein Angiography (FA) is a diagnostic technique used to evaluate the circulation of the retina and choroid.

- Purpose: To visualize the blood vessels of the retina and choroid using fluorescein dye.
- Dye used: Sodium fluorescein is injected intravenously, and a retinal fundus camera equipped with both excitation and barrier filtration captures the fluorescence.
- As the dye circulates through the retinal and choroidal vasculature, it emits a greenish-yellow fluorescence when exposed to blue excitation light, allowing the visualization of blood flow, leakage, and blockages.
- Wavelengths:
  - Excitation Light: 465–490.
  - Fluorescence Emission: 520–530.

1. Key Stages of Fluorescein Angiography in an Adult:

   The procedure occurs in the following phases post antecubital IV injection in bolus form at approximately 1 cc per second. Factors that can alter first appearance of dye and transit times include speed of IV push, location and quality of intravenous access site, and cardiac output.

   - Choroidal flush: In a normal patient, the dye appears first in the choroid approximately 10 seconds following injection. If present, the cilio-retinal artery also starts to fill at this time point.
   - Arterial phase: The central retinal artery fills one full second after the choroid.
   - Arteriovenous phase: Complete filling of the retinal capillary bed follows the arterial phase and the retinal veins begin to fill.
   - Venous phase: Complete filling of the veins occurs approximately over the next 10 seconds with maximum vessel fluorescence occurring about 30 seconds after injection.
   - Mid-Phase/Recirculation Phase: Occurs about 2 to 4 minutes post-injection.

- Late Phase: Demonstrates the gradual elimination of dye from the retinal and choroidal vasculature. Photographs are typically captured 3 to 5 minutes after injection.

2. Key Values and Parameters:

- Fluorescein Injection Dosage: The standard dose is usually 5 mL of 10% fluorescein sodium administered intravenously, though this can vary based on patient size and clinical indication. 2.5 ml of 25% is also available.
- Imaging Duration: The typical procedure lasts about 10–15 minutes, though the imaging phase itself is usually completed within 5 minutes.

3. Complications and Contraindications:

- Adverse Reactions: Common reactions can include a metallic taste in mouth, yellowing of the skin, mild nausea, and occasionally emesis. Less frequent is urticaria. Rare but serious reactions can include anaphylaxis and seizures.
- Contraindications: History of severe allergic reactions to fluorescein, pregnancy (avoided unless absolutely necessary), or renal issues. Fluorescein sodium injection has been demonstrated to be excreted in human milk for several days following fluorescein angiography, breastfeeding should therefore be discontinued for at least 4 days, and the milk should be pumped off and discarded during this period. Pumping and proper storage of milk in advance for use post-angiography should be considered [14].

Indocyanine Green Angiography (ICGA) is a diagnostic technique used primarily to assess the choroidal circulation and provide complementary information to fluorescein angiography about the retinal and choroidal vasculature in conditions such as age-related macular degeneration, choroidal neovascularization (CNV), and other retinal pathologies. It has also been used in patients that have an allergy to sodium fluorescein dye and that are not reactive to ICG dye in an attempt to reveal information that other imaging cannot such as optical coherence tomography. ICGA uses Indocyanine Green (ICG) dye, which fluoresces when exposed to near-infrared light, offering better visualization of the choroidal vessels compared to fluorescein angiography. There are two ICGA capture methods: static, where the images are taken one after another, and high-speed where the images are recorded as a video to show flow characteristics and leakage patterns.

- Purpose: To visualize the choroidal circulation and evaluate the integrity of the choroidal vasculature.
- Dye used: Indocyanine Green (ICG), a water-soluble dye that binds to plasma proteins, allowing visualization in the choroid.
- Light Wavelengths:
  - Excitation Light: 805–830 nm.
  - Fluorescence Emission: 835–870 nm.

1. Key Stages of Indocyanine Green Angiography in a Normal Adult:

The procedure occurs in the following phases post antecubital IV injection in bolus form at approximately 1 cc per second. Factors that can alter first appearance of dye and transit times include speed of IV push, location and quality of intravenous access site, and cardiac output.

- Enters choroidal vasculature approximately 10 seconds after injection.
- Then enters the arterial phase and next the venous phase.
- Late phase imaging takes place 3–20 minutes post injection; in static ICGA, late phase images are taken up to 30 minutes post injection. In high-speed ICGA capture, the last images are typically taken between 2 and 5 minutes.

2. Key Parameters and Values:

   - Dye Dosage: The standard dose of 25 mg in a 5 ml solvent of Indocyanine Green is injected typically intravenously.
   - Injection Duration: The dye is typically injected over 5 seconds.
   - Imaging Time: A static ICGA procedure usually lasts about 10–30 minutes. A high-speed ICGA procedure most often reveals the useful information by 2–3 minutes post-injection; however, later phase still/static images can be obtained if deemed necessary.
   - Fluorescence Decay: The fluorescence of ICG fades relatively slowly compared to fluorescein, allowing a longer period of observation of the choroidal circulation if needed.

3. Adverse Reactions and Contraindications:

   - Adverse Reactions: ICG is generally well tolerated, but mild reactions like nausea, vomiting, and allergic reactions can occur. Rarely, more severe reactions like anaphylaxis or hypotension may happen.
   - Contraindications: Patients with known hypersensitivity to ICG, severe liver dysfunction, or pregnancy [15].

Tear Osmolarity refers to the concentration of dissolved particles (such as salts, proteins, and other solutes) in the tears. It is an important measure used in diagnosing and managing dry eye disease (DED) and meibomian gland dysfunction (MGD). A higher tear osmolarity indicates an imbalance in the tear film, often linked to dryness, inflammation, and damage to the ocular surface.

- Normal Osmolarity: 290–300 mOsm/L.
- Elevated Osmolarity: >308 mOsm/L: Indicates an imbalance in the tear film associated with dry eye disease.
- High Osmolarity: >320 mOsm/L: Severe dry eye disease or meibomian gland dysfunction.

Low-Level Laser Therapy (LLLT) is used in the treatment of dry eye disease and meibomian gland dysfunction (MGD) by using *low-intensity lasers* to stimulate the meibomian glands and improve tear production. The technique can also help reduce inflammation in the ocular surface

- Wavelength: 600–1000 nm
- Power output: 20–200 mW
- Energy density: 2–4 J/cm^2 (joules per square centimeter)

Wavefront Aberrometry provides a comprehensive understanding of how the eye focuses light, and it is widely used in refractive surgery, assessing visual performance, and understanding conditions such *as* astigmatism, presbyopia, or keratoconus. Wavefront aberrations can be used to guide corrective measures such as LASIK *or* PRK.

Aberration types measured in wavefront aberrometry, with normal values listed:

- Total Root Mean Square (RMS) Aberrations: <0.3 μm.
- Higher-Order Aberrations (HOAs): <0.2 μm.
- Spherical Aberration: ±0.1 to ±0.2 μm.
- Coma: <0.1 μm.
- Trefoil: <0.2 μm.
- Secondary Astigmatism: <0.1 μm.
- Astigmatism: <0.5 D.
- RMS of Higher-Order Aberrations: <0.3 μm or 0.05–0.2 μm RMS.
- Zernike Coefficients for Z4 (Coma): <0.1 μm.

Gonio-photography is a specialized imaging technique used in ophthalmology to capture images of the anterior chamber angle of the eye. This is primarily relevant in the context of glaucoma assessment but is also used to document and help in the initial evaluation and follow-up visits of patients with iris tumors to track progression. The angle is formed between the cornea and the iris, and visible structures during gonio-photography include the trabecular meshwork and the iris. There are two types, direct and indirect, and both are contact lenses. Gonioscopy is the clinical technique used to visualize the anterior chamber angle, and gonio-photography may follow gonioscopy to document findings. Some gonio lens are specifically made for gonio-photography.

The Koeppe lens allows direct gonioscopy with a 50-diopter lens placed on the eye of a supine patient using saline to bridge the gap between the lens and cornea. The examiner views the angle through a hand-held binocular microscope. The Koeppe lens magnifies ×1.5. This in combination with the ×16 magnification of the oculars provides a total magnification of 24×. There are Koeppe lenses in several sizes from infant to adult. Imaging can be achieved through the Koeppe lens with some commercially available devices such as the Retcam. Indirect gonioscopy uses mirrors at certain angles within the gonio-lens to achieve views of the trabecular meshwork, etc. Indirect gonioscopic lenses use methylcellulose as the buffer between the lens and cornea of the patient, and can be used in clinic at the slit lamp/ photo-slit lamp, after proper instillation of a corneal numbing agent.

Common Types of Gonio Lenses:

- Goldmann 1-Mirror: 59° view.
- Goldmann 3-Mirror has three views: 59, 67, 73.
- Koeppe: 1.5× magnification w/ 16× oculars = magnification of 24×.

Measurements and Values:

- Angle Measurement:
- The anterior chamber angle is typically measured in degrees.
- Normal angle: 30–45 degrees.
- Narrow angle: Less than 20 degrees—may indicate potential glaucoma risk.
- Angle Classification:
  - Open Angle: >30 degrees.
  - Narrow Angle: 20–30 degrees.
  - Closed Angle: <20 degrees.
- Trabecular Meshwork:
  - The condition and visibility of the trabecular meshwork can indicate the health of the angle. It should be well defined and visible in open angles [16].

References

1. Holladay JT. Optical biometry: principles and applications. In: Wang L, Koch DD, editors. Optical biometers and intraocular lens power calculations. 2nd ed. Cham: Springer; 2021. p. 15–38.
2. Byrne SF, Green RL. Ultrasound of the eye and orbit. 2nd ed. Philadelphia: Mosby Elsevier; 2002. p. 1–45.
3. Spaide RF, Fujimoto JG, Waheed NK, Sadda SR, Staurenghi G. Optical coherence tomography angiography. In: Spaide RF, Fujimoto JG, Waheed NK, editors. Retinal OCT angiography. Cham: Springer; 2021. p. 1–54.
4. Holder GE, Robson AG, Wilkins MR, Trip SA. Electrophysiology in ophthalmology. In: Ryan SJ, Sadda SR, Hinton DR, Schachat AP, Wilkinson CP, Wiedemann P, editors. Retina, vol. 1. 5th ed. London: Elsevier; 2013. p. 507–48.
5. McCulloch DL, Marmor MF, Brigell MG, Hamilton R, Holder GE, Tzekov R, Bach M. International Society for Clinical Electrophysiology of vision. ISCEV standard for full-field clinical electroretinography (2022 update). Doc Ophthalmol. 2022;144(3):165–77. https://doi.org/10.1007/s10633-022-09866-0.
6. Frishman LJ, Sustar M, Kremers J, McAnany JJ, Sarossy M, Tzekov R, Viswanathan S. International Society for Clinical Electrophysiology of vision. ISCEV extended protocol for the photopic negative response (PhNR) of the full-field electroretinogram. Doc Ophthalmol. 2018;136(3):207–11. https://doi.org/10.1007/s10633-018-9638-x.
7. Jackson GR, Edwards JG. A short-duration dark adaptation protocol for assessment of age-related maculopathy. J Ocul Biol Dis Infor. 2008;1(1):7–11. https://doi.org/10.1007/s12177-008-9002-1.
8. Weinreb RN, Garway-Heath DF, Leung CKS, Medeiros FA, Liebmann JM, Girkin CA, Zangwill LM. Visual fields. In: Weinreb RN, Garway-Heath DF, Leung CKS, Medeiros FA, Liebmann JM, Girkin CA, Zangwill LM, editors. Diagnosis of primary open angle glaucoma. Cham: Springer; 2022. p. 69–94.
9. Birt CM, Shuey NH, Wall M. Manual kinetic perimetry: Goldmann and tangent screen. In: Kardon RH, Trobe JD, editors. Ophthalmic Perimetry: visual field examination and interpretation. Cham: Springer; 2017. p. 87–112.
10. Okonkwo ON, Baker M, Bhootic L, Uche NJ, Ritch R, Azuamah YC, Madu N, Akano F, Okeke S, Okonkwo U, Onuoha P, Achigbu E, Ezisi C, Nwachukwu L, Olali C, Akinmoladun V, Uche JN. Normative values for microperimetry with the MP-3 microperimeter: sensitivity

thresholds and fixation stability in healthy eyes. BMC Ophthalmol. 2022;22(1):123. https://doi.org/10.1186/s12886-022-02363-4.
11. Pels E, Beekhuis WH. Corneal endothelium and specular microscopy. In: Krachmer JH, Mannis MJ, Holland EJ, editors. Cornea. 3rd ed. Philadelphia: Saunders Elsevier; 2011. p. 213–32.
12. Schatz A, Pichi F, Sarraf D. Retinal imaging. In: Finger RP, Gnavi S, Wolf-Schnurrbusch U, Wolf S, editors. Advanced ophthalmic imaging. Cham: Springer; 2019. p. 21–53.
13. Schmitz-Valckenberg S, Bindewald-Wittich A, Dolar-Szczasny J, Holz FG. Fundus autofluorescence imaging. In: Holz FG, Schmitz-Valckenberg S, Spaide RF, editors. Imaging in retinal disease. Cham: Springer; 2014. p. 137–57.
14. Flower RW. Fluorescein angiography. In: Yanoff M, Duker JS, editors. Ophthalmology. 6th ed. Philadelphia: Elsevier; 2019. p. 343–57.
15. Charbel Issa P, Schmitz-Valckenberg S, Holz FG. Indocyanine green angiography. In: Holz FG, Schmitz-Valckenberg S, Spaide RF, editors. Imaging in retinal disease. Cham: Springer; 2014. p. 159–76.
16. Ritch R, Shields MB. Gonioscopy. In: Ritch R, Shields MB, Krupin T, editors. The Glaucomas. 2nd ed. St. Louis: Mosby; 1996. p. 95–122.

Chapter 17
Emerging Ocular Imaging Technology

Recent advancements in imaging technologies have significantly improved our ability to image, record, and study the structure and function of the human eye in both clinical and research settings. These technologies offer greater resolution, speed, depth, and functional insights, which are crucial for diagnosing and understanding various ocular conditions. The following are some emerging technologies that should in time prove useful in vision science and ophthalmology.

Confocal scanning laser microscopy (CSLM) is a technology in use in some research institutions. Current use includes identifying acanthamoeba keratitis and retinal applications. Recent CSLM work shows significantly reduced corneal endothelial cell density in patients with dementia. This is an advanced imaging technique that provides high-magnification, high-resolution, three-dimensional visualization of tissues. CSLM is especially valuable in ophthalmology because it provides non-invasive imaging of the eye's microstructures and tissues, enabling diagnosis and monitoring of various diseases without the need for biopsy.

CSLM Applications in Ophthalmology

Corneal Imaging: CSLM is used to visualize the different layers of the cornea in high detail. It helps in diagnosing corneal diseases such as keratoconus, Fuchs' dystrophy, and infections.

Endothelial Cell Analysis: It allows for the assessment of corneal endothelial cells which is crucial in evaluating corneal health and detecting early signs of endothelial dysfunction.

Nerve Fiber Analysis: CSLM can image the corneal nerve fibers, aiding in the diagnosis of conditions such as neurotrophic keratopathy and diabetic neuropathy.

Contact Lens Evaluation: It is used to assess the interaction between the cornea and contact lenses, helping to optimize lens fitting and detect contact lens-induced complications.

M. P. Kelly, *Normal Values in Vision Science*,
https://doi.org/10.1007/978-3-032-18207-4_17

Ocular Surface Disorders: CSLM helps in diagnosing and monitoring ocular surface diseases such as dry eye syndrome, conjunctival disorders, and limbal stem cell deficiency.

Glaucoma: It assists in the evaluation of the optic nerve head and retinal nerve fiber layer, contributing to the diagnosis and management of glaucoma.

Uveitis: It helps in the detailed examination of the retina and choroid, providing valuable information for the diagnosis and management of uveitis.

Oncology: CSLM can be used in the evaluation of ocular tumors, such as conjunctival and corneal neoplasms, by providing high-resolution images of the tumor cells.

Challenges and Limitations of CSLM

CSLM requires contact with the cornea posing a challenge to the imager and is often uncomfortable for the patient even though topical anesthetic is required and applied prior to imaging.

Depth Penetration: CSLM has limited depth penetration, making it difficult to image deeper layers of the eye, particularly in patients with thicker corneas or those with significant pathology. There is very often a trade-off between resolution and field of view (FOV). High-resolution images are limited to small areas, which can make it challenging to assess larger structures or obtain a wide field image.

Motion Artifacts: Eye movements can introduce motion artifacts in the images.

Optical Aberrations: Variations in the cornea's refractive properties can cause optical aberrations, reducing image quality and making it harder to obtain clear, detailed images.

How CSLM Works: A laser beam is focused on a specific point within the sample. The laser provides a concentrated light source, which is crucial for high-resolution imaging. In CSLM, the use of a pinhole aperture placed in front of the detector allows only the light from the focal plane to pass, while blocking out-of-focus light from other planes and results in a sharp image of the desired focal plane/tissue. The laser is scanned across the sample/tissue often in a raster pattern. As the laser scans, it builds up an image at a particular depth. The light reflected or emitted is collected by a detector. By using a pinhole, only light from the in-focus plane reaches the detector, ensuring high contrast and high resolution. The signals collected by the detector are used to create an image. Stacking these images acquired at different depths provides a detailed 3D representation of the desired tissue.

Key Parameters for Confocal Scanning Laser Microscopy (CSLM)

Resolution	1–2 μm (lateral), 2–5 μm (axial)
Field of view	400 μm × 400 μm to 1000 μm × 1000 μm
Wavelength range	488 nm to 750 nm (depending on application)
Scan speed	400 Hz to 1000 Hz
Laser power	1–20 mW (at the sample)

Signal-to-noise ratio (SNR)	35 dB to 60 dB
Pixel dimensions	0.2 µm to 0.5 µm (lateral), 2 µm to 5 µm (axial)
Depth penetration	200 µm to 500 µm
Pixel sampling rate	512 × 512 to 1024 × 1024 pixels
Optical sectioning thickness	1 µm to 5 µm

Each of these parameters can vary depending on the specific requirements of the system and application [1].

Doppler holography is an emerging technology in vision science that can measure blood flow in the eye including the retina and choroid. This technique provides information on the velocity and patterns of blood flow.

How Doppler Holography Works The technology uses of a laser to create a detailed image/hologram of tissue. The laser beam is split into two parts: the reference beam and the object beam. The object beam is directed toward the eye, where it interacts with the tissues and blood flow within the eye. When the laser from the object beam hits moving blood cells within the blood vessels of the eye, the light is scattered. Due to the Doppler effect, the frequency of the scattered light shifts depending on the speed and direction of the blood flow. If the blood cells are moving toward the laser the frequency increases, termed "blue shift," and if they are moving away it decreases, termed "red shift." The scattered light, now containing information about the blood flow, interferes with the reference beam. This interference pattern (hologram) encodes both the amplitude and phase information of the light, recording the details of the blood flow. The interference pattern is recorded by a high-resolution sensor. Algorithms reconstruct the image of the blood flow which then provides the structural image of the tissues and the flow information. Doppler shift information in the hologram is used to calculate the velocity and direction of blood flow in the retinal and choroidal vessels over a specific time frame; these create maps of the blood flow dynamics. Doppler holography can produce 3D images of the blood flow and measurements of the flow can be extracted.

Applications in Ophthalmology Diabetic retinopathy, retinal vein occlusion, age-related macular degeneration, glaucoma, ocular ischemia, and possibly other disorders may benefit from Doppler holography. It can be used to monitor the effectiveness of treatments such as anti-VEGF therapy. Doppler holography also reveals pulsatile blood flow which corresponds with the heartbeat. In a healthy adult, these pulses should be consistent with the cardiac cycle. Normal flow patterns will show consistent movement of blood through the retinal and choroidal vessels without impediment, which might indicate a blockage or other abnormality.

Challenges and Limitations Eye movement motion artifacts can affect the accuracy of measurements and the quality of the images. Doppler holography is more effective in imaging superficial structures such as the retinal blood vessels and less useful for deeper structures such as the choroid, which can be blocked by pigment and/or existing pathology.

Key Parameters of Doppler Holography

Resolution	1–5 micrometers (μm)
Field of view	1 mm to 5 mm
Magnification	20× to 100×
Wavelength	780 nm to 830 nm
Scanning speed	100 Hz to 1 kHz
Depth penetration	0.5 mm to 2 mm
Laser power	1 mW to 10 mW
Pixel dimensions	2 μm to 5 μm
Objective lens	20× to 40×

Each of these parameters can vary depending on the specific requirements of the system and application [2].

Laser Speckle Contact Imaging (LSCI) is a noninvasive imaging technique used in ophthalmology to evaluate blood flow and perfusion in the retina and optic nerve head, helping diagnose and monitor conditions such as diabetic retinopathy, glaucoma, and retinal ischemia.

How LSCI Works A laser light is directed at the retina, the light scattered by moving particles (red blood cells) forms a speckle pattern, the camera captures this speckle pattern, and the degree of contrast in the speckle is measured. The variation in speckle contrast from the movement of red blood cells is used to calculate the relative blood flow or tissue perfusion.

Applications in Ophthalmology LSCI has been applied in ophthalmology for noninvasive, real-time monitoring of blood flow in the retina and optic nerve head, offering insights into various eye conditions.

Retinal Blood Flow Measurement LSCI is used to assess retinal blood flow and identify abnormalities, which is crucial in diseases like diabetic retinopathy, glaucoma, and retinal vein occlusion. Monitoring Glaucoma: It helps in studying the blood flow to the optic nerve head, which can be altered in glaucoma, providing additional insight beyond intraocular pressure measurements. Diabetic Retinopathy: It helps detect changes in retinal perfusion due to diabetes, a critical aspect of diagnosing and monitoring diabetic retinopathy. Assessment of Retinal Ischemia: LSCI can be used to monitor areas of reduced blood flow, particularly in retinal ischemia and vascular occlusions. Pre- and Post-Surgical Evaluation: It is useful for assessing the effects of surgeries like retinal laser photocoagulation or vitrectomy on retinal perfusion.

Key Parameters of LSCI

- Axial (Depth) Resolution: ~10–30 μm.
- Lateral (Transverse) Resolution: ~10–30 μm.
- Field of View (FoV): ~1–2 mm in diameter (depends on the system and the size of the retina region being imaged).
- Magnification: ~1× to 2× magnification for retinal imaging, depending on the system and optics.
- Laser Wavelength: 780–830 nm.
- Scanning Speed: 10–100 Hz.
- Laser Power: 1–5 mW.
- Depth Penetration: ~1–2 mm in the retina, although this can vary depending on the wavelength of the laser and the specific retinal layer being imaged.
- Pixel Size: ~2–6 μm.
- Objective Lens: 50× to 100× magnification.

These values can vary slightly depending on the specific system and the imaging setup used, but they provide a general idea of the parameters for LSCI applied to retinal imaging [3].

Adaptive Optics (AO)

Retinal cameras can utilize AO to correct for optical aberrations caused by the eye's imperfect lens and cornea. This allows for detailed visualization of photoreceptors.

How Adaptive Optics Retinal Cameras Work The process uses a wavefront sensor in measuring the distortions in the wavefront of light as it passes through the eye's optical components. To correct aberrations, AO systems use deformable mirrors that can change shape in real time. The deformable mirror adjusts its surface to counteract the wavefront distortions canceling out the imperfections. This allows the light to be refocused perfectly on the retina, providing a sharp image. The adaptive optics system is continuously adjusting the deformable mirror. This constant correction ensures that the imaging remains sharp even as small movements of the eye or changes in the optical system happen. As the aberrations are corrected the retinal camera captures high-resolution images of individual cells such as photoreceptors. AO benefits from using a large pupil. Most other imaging technologies use a small beam or sub-aperture of the pupil between 0.5 mm and 3 mm as that is the range of which aberrations are minimal. Using a larger beam the resolution improvement expected from the smaller diffraction limit is outweighed by the resolution lost to aberrations. The deformable mirror corrects these aberrations allowing achievement of sub-micron resolution in vivo. AO systems generally work only over a small FOV.

Applications of AO in Retina AO can provide cellular-level information of diseases such as age-related macular degeneration and diabetic retinopathy. AO provides more detailed images than existing retinal fundus cameras and optical coherence tomography which may lead to earlier detection of diseases and for assessing the efficacy of new treatments. The ability to resolve individual retinal cells is a significant advantage over current technology. The imaging is noninvasive.

Key Parameters for Adaptive Optics

Resolution	1–2 μm
Field of view	1 mm × 1 mm to 4 mm × 4 mm
Magnification	20× to 100×
Wavelength	780 nm to 900 nm, 400 nm to 700 nm
Scanning speed	1 Hz to 10 Hz
Depth penetration	100 μm to 300 μm
Laser power	1 mW to 10 mW
Pixel dimensions	1 μm to 3 μm
Objective lens	20× to 100×

Each of these parameters can vary depending on the specific requirements of the system and application [4].

Two-Photon and Multiphoton Microscopy

TPEM imaging that allows to TPEM is used to visualize the different layers of the retina, including photoreceptors, retinal pigment epithelium, and retinal vessels as well as visualization of the structure and function of retinal tissues. It may also prove useful in imaging the anterior segment, specifically the cornea and lens.

How TPEM Works Two-photon excitation microscopy relies on the simultaneous absorption of two lower-energy photons by a fluorescent molecule to excite it to a higher energy state. The use of near-infrared light allows deeper tissue penetration due to less scatter. Because two-photon excitation occurs only at the focal point of the laser there is very little out-of-focus light and less photobleaching to surrounding tissue. TPEM provides three-dimensional imaging allowing acquisition of detailed images such as the retinal layers.

Application in Ophthalmology Retinal Imaging: TPEM will be valuable in studying the cellular mechanisms of retinal diseases such as age-related macular degeneration and diabetic retinopathy.

Challenges and Limitations TPEM has a limited field of view: 500 by 500 microns. Prolonged imaging can lead to photobleaching of fluorescent dyes or naturally occurring fluorophores in the retina, reducing the quality of images over time and potentially leading to misinterpretation of results.

Key Parameters for Two-Photon Microscopy

Resolution	0.5–1 μm
Field of view	200 μm × 200 μm to 1 mm × 1 mm
Magnification	10× to 40×
Wavelength	700 nm to 1100 nm
Scanning speed	10 Hz to 100 Hz
Depth penetration	200 μm to 500 μm
Laser power	10 mW to 100 mW
Pixel dimensions	0.2 μm to 1 μm
Objective lens	20× to 40×

Each of these parameters can vary depending on the specific requirements of the system and application [5].

Fluorescence Lifetime Imaging Ophthalmoscopy (FLIO)

FLIO measures the fluorescence lifetime of natural fluorophores in the retina. It provides information about the metabolic state of the retinal tissues and is being explored for its potential in diagnosing retinal diseases. Unlike traditional fluorescence imaging which relies on the intensity of emitted light, FLIO captures the time it takes for excited molecules to return to their ground state after being excited by a light source. This time interval (fluorescence lifetime) provides information about the molecular environment and can be used to study metabolic processes in the retina.

How FLIO Works When a fluorophore absorbs light it excites and eventually returns to its ground state, emitting light in the process. The time between excitation and emission, measured in nanoseconds, is known as the fluorescence lifetime. FLIO typically uses a technique called time-correlated single photon counting (TCSPC) to measure the fluorescence lifetime. A pulsed laser excites the fluorophores in the retina and detectors capture the emitted photons. The time delay between the excitation pulse and the detected photon is recorded and the fluorescence lifetime is calculated from these measurements. FLIO can detect changes in the metabolic state of retinal tissues by analyzing variations in fluorescence lifetime. This is useful for studying diseases that alter the metabolic environment of the retina, for example, age-related macular degeneration, diabetic retinopathy, and retinal dystrophies. It primarily detects the fluorescence of naturally occurring fluorophores in the retina, such as lipofuscin which is a by-product of photoreceptor degradation. The fluorescence lifetime of these molecules seem to provide useful information about the retinal disease state in some disorders.

Applications in Ophthalmology: FLIO can detect early changes in the retina associated with AMD prior to them appearing on traditional retinal imaging. Changes in fluorescence lifetime can indicate oxidative stress or the accumulation of toxic by-products. It may also help to identify early metabolic changes in the retina caused by the diabetic state, allowing for earlier intervention. FLIO may be useful with inherited retinal dystrophies by providing "metabolic-fingerprints," and in determining the efficacy of gene therapy treatments.

Challenges and Limitations Fluorescence lifetimes can vary between individuals, and this may pose challenging to establishing reference values. FLIO is mostly used to image the retinal pigment epithelium or photoreceptors. Because of the limited penetration of the excitation, light it is not as effective in imaging the choroid.

Key Parameters for FLIO

Resolution	10–20 μm
Field of view	30° to 50° (5 mm × 5 mm to 10 mm × 10 mm)
Magnification	1.5× to 3×
Wavelength	Excitation: 480 nm to 490 nm; emission: 500 nm to 650 nm
Scanning speed	1 Hz to 10 Hz
Depth penetration	100 μm to 200 μm
Laser power	0.1 mW to 10 mW
Pixel dimensions	1 μm to 10 μm
Objective lens	20× to 40×

Each of these parameters can vary depending on the specific requirements of the system and application [6].

Hyperspectral Imaging (HSI)

Hyperspectral imaging (HSI) captures a wide spectrum of light providing information about the biochemical composition of tissues. It is an advanced imaging technology that captures and processes information across the electromagnetic spectrum, providing insight into the structural and the biochemical properties of the retina and other tissues.

How Hyperspectral Imaging Works Traditional imaging captures images in three color channels: red, green, and blue. HSI captures light in many spectral bands from UV through the visible spectrum, into the near-infrared creating a 3D hyperspectral cube.

Applications in Ophthalmology HSI may increase early detection early of diabetic retinopathy, age-related macular degeneration, and glaucoma, and to possibly assess the efficacy of treatments such as anti-VEGF therapy. It may also help characterize inherited retinal dystrophies through identification of "spectral fingerprints" associated with different genetic mutations.

Key Parameters for Hyperspectral Imaging

Resolution	2–10 μm
Field of view	5 mm × 5 mm to 15 mm × 15 mm
Spectral range	400 nm to 1000 nm
Spectral resolution	5 nm to 20 nm
Scanning speed	1 Hz to 10 Hz
Depth penetration	200 μm to 500 μm
Laser power	1 mW to 10 mW
Pixel dimensions	1 μm to 5 μm
Objective lens	20× to 50×

Each of these parameters can vary depending on the specific requirements of the system and application [7, 8].

Optical Coherence Tomography Elastography (OCTE)

OCTE is an emerging technology that combines OCT with elastography, which measures tissue stiffness. It is an advanced imaging technology that combines the high-resolution structural imaging capabilities of optical coherence tomography (OCT) with the ability to measure the mechanical properties of tissues. OCTE is emerging as a tool for assessing the biomechanical properties of the cornea, retina, and other ocular tissues. This can be useful in assessing biomechanical properties of the cornea and sclera possibly assisting in the diagnosis of glaucoma and/or keratoconus and other corneal disorders. Its ability to measure tissue stiffness and elasticity offers new diagnostic possibilities.

How OCT Elastography (OCTE) Works Elastography involves applying a mechanical force such as an air puff, sound waves, or direct mechanical compression to the tissue and then measuring the resulting deformation. In static elastography, the tissue is subjected to a steady or varying pressure. Dynamic methods involve applying a time-varying force, such as an acoustic wave, to induce oscillations or waves in the tissue. OCT is then used to track these waves.

Applications in Ophthalmology OCTE is useful in evaluating the mechanical properties of the cornea in conditions keratoconus and in preoperative assessment for refractive surgery. The stiffness of the optic nerve head and surrounding tissues may be linked to the development and progression of glaucoma. The changes in mechanical properties of the retina may occur in diseases such as age-related macular degeneration and OCTE may provide additional information at various stages of the disorder.

Key Parameters for OCTE

Resolution	3–5 μm
Field of view	6 mm × 6 mm to 10 mm × 10 mm
Scanning speed	20,000 to 100,000 A-scans per second
Depth penetration	1 mm to 3 mm
Laser wavelength	800 nm to 860 nm
A-scan resolution	1 to 3 μm
B-scan frame rate	30 Hz to 100 Hz
Optical power	1 mW to 5 mW
Signal-to-noise ratio	90 dB to 100 dB
Objective lens	30× to 50×

Each of these parameters can vary depending on the specific requirements of the system and application [9, 10].

Photoacoustic Imaging (PAI)

PAI is an imaging technique that combines laser-induced ultrasound with optical imaging, resulting in high-resolution images of ocular tissues and vasculature. It aims to reveal blood flow and tissue oxygenation in the retina and choroid through the combination of optical and ultrasonic imaging.

How Photoacoustic Imaging (PAI) Works PAI is based on the photoacoustic effect where short pulses of laser light are absorbed by tissues causing a rapid thermal expansion and generating ultrasonic waves. These waves are then detected by ultrasound transducers and used to create detailed images of the tissue structure. It is able to resolve fine details of blood vessels and layers of the retina. Different tissues absorb light at specific wavelengths providing the information for PAI to elicit oxygen saturation levels in blood vessels.

Applications in Ophthalmology PAI may be particularly valuable in diagnosing and monitoring diabetic retinopathy, age-related macular degeneration (AMD), and glaucoma and may help in the detection and of ocular tumors, such as choroidal melanoma. It may also provide insights into the metabolic activity of the retina.

Challenges The highly scattering tissues of the retina can compromise the optical resolution of PAI resulting in lower image quality in some cases. Achieving high resolution at greater depths remains a technical challenge. PAI imaging is susceptible to noise and artifacts mostly due to highly reflective structures, i.e., optic nerve head. Safety considerations may need to be overcome to allow widespread use.

Key Parameters for Photoacoustic Imaging

Resolution	20–100 μm
Field of view	2 mm × 2 mm to 10 mm × 10 mm
Wavelength range	700 nm to 900 nm
Depth penetration	1 mm to 3 mm
Scanning speed	1 Hz to 10 Hz
Laser power	10 mW to 100 mW
Signal-to-noise ratio	40 dB to 60 dB
Ultrasound frequency	10 MHz to 40 MHz
Pixel dimensions	10 μm to 50 μm
Objective lens	20× to 40×

Each of these parameters can vary depending on the specific requirements of the system and application [11, 12].

Retinal Densitometry

This technology allows for the assessment of retinal function of the photoreceptors, providing valuable insights into retinal diseases and conditions. Retinal Densitometry is a specialized imaging technique used to measure the density and distribution of photopigments in the retina.

How Retinal Densitometry Works The technology is based on the principle that photopigments in the retina absorb light at specific wavelengths. By measuring the changes in light absorption after the retina is exposed to light, retinal densitometry can quantify the amount of photopigment present. First, the retina is exposed to light to "bleach" the photopigments, reducing their concentration. Next, the retina is allowed to dark-adapt, during which the photopigments regenerate. Densitometry measures the rate and extent of this regeneration allowing information about the photoreceptor function. Retinal densitometry requires imaging of the retina at different time-points during and after light exposure. These images are analyzed to determine the density of photopigments by comparing the absorption of light before and after the bleaching. Specific wavelengths of light are used to target the absorption spectra of various photopigments.

Applications in Ophthalmology By measuring how quickly and effectively photopigments regenerate after bleaching, one can detect dysfunctions that may not be visible with standard imaging techniques. Early changes in retinal diseases such as retinitis pigmentosa (RP), age-related macular degeneration (AMD), and retinal dystrophies may benefit from this technology. In patients with known retinal conditions, retinal densitometry may also be useful in monitoring disease progression and the effectiveness of gene therapy and other types of interventions.

Challenges and Limitations Variability in light exposure can lead to inaccurate measurements and make it difficult to compare results visit to visit or between patients. Fluctuations in the device can introduce noise or artifacts affecting measurements and accuracy.

Key Parameters for Retinal Densitometry

Resolution	10–20 μm
Field of view	30° to 50° (~6 mm to 10 mm diameter)
Wavelength range	400 nm–520 nm
Measurement units	Optical density (OD)
Scan duration	2–5 seconds per scan
Pixel dimensions	10 μm to 2 μm
Signal-to-noise ratio	40 dB to 60 dB
Macular pigment optical density (MPOD)	0.2 to 0.7
Foveal densitometry	0.3–0.5 OD at fovea
Retinal pigment epithelium density	0.2–0.6 OD
Choroidal density	0.2–0.8 OD

Each of these parameters can vary depending on the specific requirements of the system and application [13–16].

Full-Field Optical Coherence Tomography (FF-OCT)

FF-OCT provides a wider field of view at a single depth plane, while OCT provides a detailed cross-sectional view of the tissue at a specific location. FF-OCT enables *en face* views at a given depth with subcellular resolution. OCT uses a focused beam to scan across the tissue, building a three-dimensional image by taking multiple cross sections. FF-OCT does not require lateral scanning, as the entire field of view is captured at once. FF-OCT is superior to OCT in speed and in resolution. Recent work has been exploring the use of *swept-source* FF-OCT.

How Full-Field Optical Coherence Tomography Works Conventional OCT uses a scanning method to acquire images one slice at a time; FF-OCT acquires full-field images in a single capture. This is achieved by illuminating the entire area of interest with a broad-spectrum light source and then capturing the reflected light to create a detailed image. The reflected light is detected by a sensor and the data processed to create high-resolution cross-sectional images.

Applications in Ophthalmology FF-OCT can be used to diagnose and monitor retinal diseases such as macular degeneration, diabetic retinopathy, and retinal vein occlusion. It can also be used to visualize the cornea and anterior chamber, which may be valuable for assessing anterior segment abnormalities. It may also help in assessing the optic nerve head and nerve fiber layers in glaucoma.

Challenges and Limitations FF-OCT depth penetration is limited in comparison to some other imaging modalities affecting its ability to resolve deeper structures, and images can be affected by motion artifacts.

Key Parameters for FF-OCT

Resolution	3 μm axial, 15 um lateral
Field of view	5 mm × 5 mm to 15 mm × 15 mm
Magnification	20× to 50×
Wavelength	800 nm to 1300 nm (NIR)
Scanning speed	1 Hz to 100 Hz
Depth penetration	1 mm to 3 mm
Laser power	1 mW to 10 mW
Pixel dimensions	2 μm to 5 μm
Objective lens	10× to 50×
[17–20]	

References

1. Gao N, Simpson TL. Confocal microscopy in ophthalmology: current status and future prospects. In: Holz FG, Schmitz-Valckenberg S, Spaide RF, editors. Imaging in retinal disease. Cham: Springer; 2014. p. 215–37.
2. Li X, Picart P, Dubois A. Doppler holography for quantitative blood flow imaging in the eye. In: Schmitz-Valckenberg S, Holz FG, Spaide RF, editors. Imaging in retinal disease. Cham: Springer; 2014. p. 189–203.
3. Briers JD, Webster S. Laser speckle contrast imaging for measuring blood flow. In: Schmitz-Valckenberg S, Holz FG, Spaide RF, editors. Imaging in retinal disease. Cham: Springer; 2014. p. 205–20.
4. Roorda A. Adaptive optics for studying visual function: a comprehensive review. In: Chalupa LM, Werner JS, editors. The visual neurosciences. 2nd ed. Cambridge, MA: MIT Press; 2004. p. 1203–15.
5. Masters BR. Multiphoton excitation fluorescence microscopy and confocal microscopy imaging of human ocular tissue. J Microsc. 2011;242(2):123–37. https://doi.org/10.1111/j.1365-2818.2010.03461.x.
6. Schmitz-Valckenberg S, Sauer L, Fleckenstein M, Holz FG. Fluorescence lifetime imaging ophthalmoscopy (FLIO) in ophthalmology. Prog Retin Eye Res. 2020;76:100801. https://doi.org/10.1016/j.preteyeres.2020.100801.
7. Lu G, Fei B. Medical hyperspectral imaging: a review. J Biomed Opt. 2014;19(1):010901. https://doi.org/10.1117/1.JBO.19.1.010901.
8. Sujatha N, Dhanasekaran R, Subramanian KK. Hyperspectral imaging in retinal diseases: current status and future perspectives. Surv Ophthalmol. 2022;67(3):450–64. https://doi.org/10.1016/j.survophthal.2021.11.006.
9. Wang J, Bi Q, Wang X, et al. Optical coherence elastography in ocular biomechanics: a review. Prog Retin Eye Res. 2022;88:101007. https://doi.org/10.1016/j.preteyeres.2022.101007.
10. Kennedy BF, Lee WS, Sampson DD. Elastography in ophthalmology: technologies and clinical applications. Prog Retin Eye Res. 2017;60:101–31. https://doi.org/10.1016/j.preteyeres.2017.03.003.

11. Liu C, Zhang Y, Yao J. Photoacoustic imaging in ophthalmology. Prog Retin Eye Res. 2021;80:100870. https://doi.org/10.1016/j.preteyeres.2020.100870.
12. Huang S, Zhang Y, Wang L, et al. Advances in photoacoustic imaging for ophthalmic applications. J Biophotonics. 2022;15(4):e202100234. https://doi.org/10.1002/jbio.202100234.
13. Delori FC. Spectral reflectance and transmittance of the human ocular fundus. Invest Ophthalmol Vis Sci. 1983;24(6):711–7.
14. Dorey CK, Vingrys AJ. Retinal densitometry: fundamentals and clinical applications. In: Osborne NN, Chader GJ, editors. Progress in retinal research. Amsterdam: Elsevier; 1993. p. 1–30.
15. Snodderly DM, Auran JD, Delori FC. The macular pigment. II. Spatial distribution in primate retinas. Invest Ophthalmol Vis Sci. 1984;25(6):674–85.
16. Holz FG, Schutt F, Ehrhardt C, et al. Quantitative fundus autofluorescence and retinal densitometry in age-related macular degeneration. Retina. 2010;30(9):1475–81.
17. Dubois A, Vabre L, Boccara AC, Beaurepaire E, Cazaux F, Saint-Jalmes H, et al. High-resolution full-field optical coherence tomography with a Linnik microscope. Appl Opt. 2002;41(4):805–12.
18. Leitgeb RA, Hitzenberger CK, Fercher AF. Performance of Fourier domain vs. time domain optical coherence tomography. Opt Express. 2003;11(8):889–94.
19. Schmitt JM. Optical coherence tomography (OCT): a review. IEEE J Sel Top Quantum Electron. 1999;5(4):1205–15.
20. Labin AC, Huard D, Arbel D. Functional full-field optical coherence tomography: a new tool for retinal imaging. Prog Retin Eye Res. 2020;75:100804.

Chapter 18
Future Directions

Reference measurements obtained from healthy populations (normative values) are foundational tools in ophthalmology and vision science. These benchmarks enable clinicians to detect deviations indicative of disease and to monitor progression over time. As technology, data science, predictive and personalized medicine advance, the application of normative data is poised to become even more precise and integrated. The full potential of emerging directions for normative databases and their expanding role in both clinical and research domains may have yet to be fully realized. Equally robust normative databases for children are still needed, as most initial efforts have focused primarily on adults. Regulatory bodies and manufacturers must coordinate to achieve standardization across platforms. And longitudinal studies are needed to assess how normal values shift with age and environmental factors.

Precision Ophthalmology

- Trend: Moving from one-size-fits-all reference ranges to individualized baselines.
- Impact: Allows for detecting subtle deviations from a patient's own norm, rather than just from population averages.
- Example: Tracking changes in retinal nerve fiber layer (RNFL) thickness over time using personalized longitudinal data.

Integration of Genomic and Demographic Data

- Trend: Normative databases will incorporate genetic, ethnic, and demographic variables.

M. P. Kelly, *Normal Values in Vision Science*,
https://doi.org/10.1007/978-3-032-18207-4_18

- Impact: Enhances accuracy in detecting disease, especially in diverse populations where ocular measurements can vary significantly.
- Example: Tailoring glaucoma risk assessments by combining IOP norms with ancestry-specific optic disc size data.

Population-Specific and Global Databases

- Trend: Development of regional and global normative datasets.
- Impact: Improves diagnostic accuracy in underrepresented populations.
- Example: Building separate normative data for indigenous, African, and Asian populations using OCT and visual field testing.

Longitudinal Normative Databases

- Trend: Shifting from static norms to age-adjusted, time-series data.
- Impact: Better tracking of progressive diseases.
- Example: Creating patient-specific progression curves to detect pathologic change earlier than population-based thresholds.

Multi-Modality Integration

- Trend: Combining normative data from multiple imaging and functional platforms (OCT, FAF, ERG, VF, etc.).
- Impact: Supports more holistic, system-level assessments of ocular health.
- Example: Integrating RNFL thickness, macular sensitivity, and electrophysiologic function to stratify glaucoma risk.

Normative Data in Virtual and Tele-Ophthalmology

- Trend: Expanding normative databases for remote screening tools and home-based diagnostics.
- Impact: Increases accessibility and accuracy of remote eye care.
- Example: Using normative contrast sensitivity and Amsler grid response ranges for monitoring AMD from home.

Integration into Clinical Decision Support Systems

- Trend: Embedding normative data into electronic health records (EHRs) and diagnostic platforms.
- Impact: Enables real-time alerts for abnormal findings, improving workflow and decision-making.
- Example: Automated flags in OCT software when a value falls outside the age- and race-adjusted norm.

AI-Driven Normative Modeling

- Trend: Use of machine learning to create dynamic, multidimensional normative models.
- Impact: Enables real-time identification of abnormal patterns in complex imaging and functional datasets.
- Example: AI analyzing OCT volumes and comparing them to large-scale normative databases for early detection of subclinical disease.

Artificial intelligence systems are inherently limited by the quality of the data on which they are trained. As healthcare advances toward precision medicine and the integration of augmented intelligence, recent research continues to affirm a long-standing axiom: garbage in, garbage out. In medical imaging, particularly ophthalmology, the consequences of suboptimal data are significant. Inaccurately labeled or low-resolution images not only impair model performance but also contribute to hidden stratification, a phenomenon wherein models that perform adequately on aggregate fail to generalize across specific and often vulnerable subpopulations. These failures are not mere statistical anomalies but represent meaningful clinical risks. Robust model development requires the inclusion of both diseased and normal imaging data to ensure comprehensive representation of diagnostic variation. The underrepresentation of either can skew learning, impair model calibration, and limit clinical applicability. It has been shown that the exclusion of low-value or noisy data can enhance model robustness. Valuation frameworks can provide standardized assessments of medical imaging datasets, emphasizing critical metrics such as accuracy and completeness to promote the development of trustworthy artificial intelligence systems. In ophthalmology, where diagnostic precision can depend on micron-level variations, image fidelity is essential. High-resolution, clinically validated imaging must form the basis of any AI model intended for clinical deployment. The future of medical AI will be shaped by rigorous curation and validation of the data on which these systems rely.

The future uses of normative values in ophthalmology and vision science lies in precision, inclusivity, and integration. As normative databases grow in depth and sophistication, they will become increasingly central to early diagnosis, disease monitoring, and the customization of care in both clinical and research settings. Personalized and predictive medicine is poised to benefit from digital twin technology and Big-AI in the surgical ophthalmology realm [1–8].

Of Related Interest: Digital Twin Technology

Iliuţă ME, Moisescu MA, Caramihai SI, Cernian A, Pop E, Chiş DI, Mitulescu TC. Digital twin models for personalized and predictive medicine in ophthalmology. Technologies. 2024;12:55. https://doi.org/10.3390/technologies12040055.

References

1. Wang M, Medeiros FA, Zangwill LM, et al. Longitudinal analysis of retinal nerve fiber layer thickness for glaucoma progression. Ophthalmology. 2013;120(2):249–57.
2. Varma R, Ying-Lai M, Francis BA, et al. Race-, ethnicity-, and ancestry-based differences in intraocular pressure and optic disc morphology. Arch Ophthalmol. 2011;129(3):301–8.
3. De Fauw J, Keane PA, Tomasev K, et al. Clinically applicable deep learning for diagnosis and referral in retinal disease. Nat Med. 2018;24(9):1342–50.
4. Tham YC, Li X, Wong TY, et al. Global prevalence of glaucoma and projections of glaucoma burden through 2040. Ophthalmology. 2014;121(11):2081–90.
5. Wu Z, Lee J, Lee CS, et al. Longitudinal changes in optical coherence tomography measurements for glaucoma detection. Am J Ophthalmol. 2019;200:162–72.
6. Baniasadi N, Lee CS, Lee AY, et al. Multimodal data integration in ophthalmology: challenges and future directions. Front Med (Lausanne). 2021;8:713768.
7. Sommer A. The promise and challenge of tele-ophthalmology. JAMA Ophthalmol. 2020;138(9):877–8.
8. Schmidt-Erfurth U, Sadeghipour A, Gerendas BS, et al. Artificial intelligence in retina: the future is here. Ophthalmol Retina. 2022;6(4):339–49.

Appendix A: Key Measurement Terms and Their Abbreviations in Ophthalmology and Vision Science

General Measurements:

IOP: Intraocular Pressure (measured in millimeters of mercury, mm Hg).
CCT: Central Corneal Thickness (measured in microns, µm).
ACD: Anterior Chamber Depth (measured in millimeters, mm).
AL: Axial Length (measured in millimeters, mm).
CMT: Central Macular Thickness (measured in microns, µm).
RNFL: Retinal Nerve Fiber Layer (measured in microns, µm).
BCVA: Best-Corrected Visual Acuity (e.g., 20/20 or 6/6 or 1.0 decimal).
VA: Visual Acuity (e.g., 20/20 or 6/6 or 1.0 decimal).
CDR: Cup-to-Disc Ratio (expressed as a decimal, e.g., 0.3).
K: Keratometry (curvature of the cornea measured in diopters, D).
PD: Pupillary Distance (measured in millimeters, mm).
TBUT: Tear Film Break-Up Time (measured in seconds, s).
FAZ: Foveal Avascular Zone (measured in microns, µm or in millimeters, mm).
OPA: Ocular pulse amplitude (measured in mm Hg).
Arc-seconds, indicated as: "(double prime symbol). In use, i.e.,: 5".

[1–10].

Refractive Measurements:

D: Diopters (unit of refractive power).
Sph: Spherical (measured in diopters, D).
Cyl: Cylinder (measured in diopters, D).

M. P. Kelly, *Normal Values in Vision Science*,
https://doi.org/10.1007/978-3-032-18207-4

Axis: Axis of astigmatism (measured in degrees, °).
ADD: Addition (measured in diopters, D).
MRSE: Mean Refractive Spherical Equivalent (measured in diopters, D).

[11–14].

Appendix B: Key Units of Measurement and Their Abbreviations in Vision Science and Ophthalmology

Flow Velocities

- cm/s—Centimeters per second
- mm/s—Millimeters per second
- m/s—Meters per second

Weights

- mg—Milligrams
- g—Grams
- kg—Kilograms

Degrees (Angles)

- °—Degrees
- Δ (Prism Diopters)—Measurement of prismatic power in eyeglasses

Volumes

- μL—Microliters
- mL—Milliliters
- L—Liters

Liquid Volumes

- mL/min—Milliliters per minute
- μL/min—Microliters per minute

Refractive Powers

- D (Diopter)—Unit of measure for the optical power of lenses
- PD (Pupillary Distance)—Measured in millimeters

Indexes

- n (Refractive Index)—Dimensionless number indicating how light propagates through a medium
- IOP (Intraocular Pressure)—Measured in mmHg (millimeters of mercury)
- RI (Retinal Index)—Used in specialized retinal imaging

M. P. Kelly, *Normal Values in Vision Science*,
https://doi.org/10.1007/978-3-032-18207-4

Rates and Speeds
- Hz (Hertz)—Cycles per second, used for frequency
- cpm (Cycles per minute)—Used for blinking or other repetitive ocular actions
- mm/min—Millimeters per minute, e.g., for tear production rate (Schirmer test)

Degrees per Second
- °/s—Degrees per second, used to measure eye movement velocity

Densities
- g/cm^3—Grams per cubic centimeter, used in measuring lens material density

Pressures
- mmHg (millimeters of mercury)—Used for intraocular pressure (IOP) measurements

Optical Characteristics
- Abbe number—Dimensionless number indicating the dispersion of a lens material
- UV Transmission—Percentage of ultraviolet light transmitted through a lens

Blood Flow and Oxygen Measurements
- µm/s (Microns or Micrometers per second)—Used to measure retinal blood flow velocity
- % O2 (Oxygen Saturation)—Percentage used to measure blood oxygen in retinal vessels
- SvO_2—oxygen saturation in retinal veins
- SaO_2—oxygen saturation in retinal arteries

Photometry
- cd/m^2 (Candela per Square Meter)—Luminance, used in visual field testing and brightness measurements
- lx (Lux)—Illuminance, used to measure light levels in visual environments
- lm (Lumen)—Used to measure the luminous flux of light sources
- mJ (millijoules)—Energy delivered in laser treatments
- ns (nanoseconds)—Measure of duration of nanosecond pulsed lasers
- fs (femtoseconds)—Measure of ultrafast laser pulses
- mW (milliwatts)—Measure of the power of light sources

Time-Related Measurements
- ms (Milliseconds)—Used for measuring reaction times, latency, or visual processing speed

Spatial Frequency
- cpd (Cycles per Degree)—Used to measure contrast sensitivity or spatial resolution

Field of View
- dpt (Diopters per Meter)—Used for visual acuity measurements related to lens power

Corneal Curvature and Thickness

- mm (Millimeters)—Used for corneal curvature (keratometry) and axial length measurements
- μm (Microns or micrometers)—Used for measuring corneal and retinal thickness

Spectral Sensitivity

- nm (Nanometers)—Used to measure wavelengths of light, relevant for color vision and photoreceptor sensitivity

Accommodative and Vergence Measurements

- MA (Meter Angle)—Used to measure convergence and divergence in binocular vision testing
- AA (Amplitude of Accommodation)—Measured in diopters (D)

Pupil Measurements

- mm (Millimeters)—Used to measure pupil diameter

Photopic and Scotopic Conditions

- cd/m^2 (Candela per Square Meter)—Photopic conditions
- mcd/m^2 (Millicandela per Square Meter)—Scotopic conditions

Optical Density

- OD (Optical Density)—Dimensionless unit used to measure the attenuation of light

Appendix C: Units of Measure (Alphabetical)

Unit/ symbol	Full name/description	Typical use in ophthalmology
AA	Amplitude of accommodation	Measurement of near-focusing ability
cd/m^2	Candela per square meter	Luminance of light sources or stimuli
$cd{\cdot}s/m^2$	Candela·seconds per square meter	Light stimulus intensity in ERG
cm/s	Centimeters per second	Eye movement or blood flow velocity
cpd	Cycles per degree	Spatial frequency in vision testing
$cpd/deg.^2$	Cycles per degree squared	Microperimetry or detailed spatial mapping
cpm	Cycles per minute	Slow oscillations, eye tracking
Δ	Prism diopters	Measurement of ocular deviation
dpt	Diopters per meter	Lens power or optical vergence
°	Degrees	Angles of gaze, visual field, or fixation
°/s	Degrees per second	Eye movement velocity (saccades, pursuit)
FOV °	Field of view in degrees	Visual field assessment
g	Grams	Mass of ocular structures in research
g/cm^3	Grams per cubic centimeter	Density of tissues or fluids
Hz	Hertz	Frequency of flicker stimuli or oscillations
I	Intensity	Light stimulus or reflectance
kg	Kilograms	Rarely used; overall ocular mass research
L	Liters	Volume of aqueous or vitreous humor in large-scale models
lm	Lumen	Photometric output of light sources
lux (lx)	Illuminance	Ambient light level or stimulus exposure
lux·s	Lux-seconds	Light exposure dose (phototoxicity or experimental)
logMAR	Logarithm of minimum angle of resolution	Standardized visual acuity scale
MA	Meter angle	Ocular angular measurement in optics

M. P. Kelly, *Normal Values in Vision Science*,
https://doi.org/10.1007/978-3-032-18207-4

Unit/ symbol	Full name/description	Typical use in ophthalmology
mcd/m^2	Millicandela per square meter	Low-luminance stimuli
mg	Milligrams	Small mass measurements of tissues or implants
mL	Milliliters	Volume of ocular fluids
mL/min	Milliliters per minute	Aqueous humor production rate
mm	Millimeters	Axial length, corneal thickness, etc.
mmHg	Millimeters of mercury	Intraocular or perfusion pressure
mm/min	Millimeters per minute	Slow movement measurements (e.g., vascular flow)
mm/s	Millimeters per second	Flow velocity in vessels or ocular movement
MPa	Megapascals	Pressure measurements in corneal biomechanics
ms	Milliseconds	Timing in electrophysiology (ERG, VEP)
$nV/deg.^2$	Nanovolts per degree squared	Multifocal ERG response amplitude
nm	Nanometers	Wavelength of light stimuli or imaging
OD	Optical density	Absorbance or filter characterization
Pa	Pascals	Alternative unit for intraocular or perfusion pressure
$Cells/mm^2$	Cells per square millimeter	Corneal endothelial cell density
μL	Microliters	Small fluid volumes (aqueous, tears)
μL/min	Microliters per minute	Micro-scale flow rates
μm	Micrometers	Tissue thickness, retinal layers, cornea
μm^3	Cubic microns	Tissue or cellular volume in histology
μm/s	Microns per second	Micro-scale flow velocity or movement
μV	Microvolts	ERG, VEP, EOG signal amplitude
mOsm/kg	Milliosmoles per kilogram	Osmolarity of tears or aqueous humor
% O_2	Oxygen saturation	Retinal or tissue oxygenation
Td	Trolands	Retinal illuminance (luminance × pupil area)
VA fraction	Visual acuity fraction	Snellen fraction (e.g., 20/20)
W/m^2	Watts per square meter	Light irradiance or phototherapy
ΔL or ΔT	Change in luminance or transmittance	Contrast sensitivity testing

Appendix D: Key Units of Measure (Grouped by Unit Type)

Vision & Optics

- AA—amplitude of accommodation.
- Abbe number—chromatic dispersion.
- cpd—cycles per Degree,
- Δ—prism diopters.
- dpt—diopters per meter,
- MA—meter angle.
- OD—optical density.

Light & Illumination

- cd/m^2—candela per square meter,
- mcd/m^2—millicandela per square meter,
- lm—lumen,
- l× (Lux)—illuminance.

Mass & Density

- g—grams,
- mg—milligrams,
- kg—kilograms,
- g/cm^3—grams per cubic centimeter.

Length & Distance

- mm—millimeters,
- μm—microns or micrometers,
- nm—nanometers.

Volume & Flow

- L—liters.
- mL—milliliters,
- μL—microliters,

M. P. Kelly, *Normal Values in Vision Science*,
https://doi.org/10.1007/978-3-032-18207-4

- mL/min—milliliters per minute,
- μL/min—microliters per minute.

Pressure
- mmHg—millimeters of mercury,
- MPa—megapascals.

Speed & Velocity
- cm/s—centimeters per second,
- mm/s—millimeters per second,
- μm/s—microns or micrometers per second,
- m/s—meters per second.

Time & Frequency
- Hz—hertz.
- cpm—cycles per minute,
- ms—milliseconds.

Angle & Motion
- °—degrees
- °/s—degrees per second.

Other
- % O2—oxygen saturation.

Appendix E: Comparative Measurements of Ocular Structures

Diameter

- Anterior Chamber: N/A.
- Aqueous Humor: N/A.
- Choroid: N/A (surrounds retina, size like sclera).
- Cornea: 11.5–12 mm.
- Lens: 9–10 mm.
- Optic Nerve: 3–4 mm.
- Retina: 22 mm (diameter of the entire retina).
- Sclera: N/A (forms outer shell).
- Vitreous Body: N/A (fills posterior chamber).

Depth

- Anterior Chamber: 3–4 mm.
- Aqueous Humor: N/A (fills anterior chamber).
- Choroid: 0.2–0.5 mm.
- Cornea: 0.5–0.6 mm (central), 0.7 mm (peripheral).
- Lens: 4–5 mm.
- Optic Nerve: N/A.
- Retina: 0.1–0.5 mm.
- Sclera: 0.3–1.0 mm.
- Vitreous Body: N/A (fills the chamber).

Density

- Anterior Chamber: 1.0 g/cm^3.
- Aqueous Humor: 1.0 g/cm^3.
- Choroid: 1.06 g/cm^3 (due to blood vessels).
- Cornea: 1.05 g/cm^3.
- Lens: 1.1 g/cm^3.
- Optic Nerve: 1.05 g/cm^3.

M. P. Kelly, *Normal Values in Vision Science*,
https://doi.org/10.1007/978-3-032-18207-4

- Retina: 1.05 g/cm^3 (varies by layer).
- Sclera: 1.35 g/cm^3.
- Vitreous Body: 1.02 g/cm^3.

Pressure
- Anterior Chamber: Intraocular pressure (10–21 mmHg).
- Aqueous Humor: Contributes to intraocular pressure.
- Choroid: N/A (helps in blood supply).
- Cornea: N/A (affected by intraocular pressure).
- Lens: N/A.
- Optic Nerve: N/A.
- Retina: N/A.
- Sclera: N/A.
- Vitreous Body: Affects intraocular pressure.

Stiffness
- Anterior Chamber: N/A.
- Aqueous Humor: N/A.
- Choroid: 0.05–0.1 MPa (similar to soft tissue).
- Cornea: Approx. 0.1–0.2 MPa.
- Lens: Low (stiffens with age).
- Optic Nerve: Relatively soft tissue.
- Retina: Soft tissue (varies with pathology).
- Sclera: 0.5–0.9 MPa.
- Vitreous Body: Viscoelastic (gel-like).

Thickness
- Anterior Chamber: N/A (depth varies with individual).
- Aqueous Humor: N/A (fills anterior chamber).
- Choroid: 0.2–0.5 mm (varies with location).
- Cornea: 0.5–0.6 mm (central), 0.7 mm (peripheral).
- Lens: 4–5 mm.
- Optic Nerve: 3–4 mm.
- Retina: 0.1–0.5 mm (varies across regions).
- Sclera: 0.3–1.0 mm.
- Vitreous Body: N/A (fills the chamber).

Volume
- Anterior Chamber: 0.25–0.3 mL.
- Aqueous Humor: 0.3 mL.
- Choroid: 4–6 mL.
- Cornea: 0.2–0.3 mL.
- Lens: 0.5–1.0 mL.
- Optic Nerve: 0.5–1 mL.
- Retina: 1–1.5 mL.
- Sclera: 16–18 mL.
- Vitreous Body: 4–5 mL.

Weight

- Anterior Chamber: N/A.
- Aqueous Humor: 0.3 g.
- Choroid: 0.2–0.3 g (wet), 0.04–0.06 g (dry).
- Cornea: 0.5–0.55 g (wet), 0.09–0.12 g (dry).
- Lens: 0.17–0.25 g (wet), 0.08–0.12 g (dry).
- Optic Nerve: 0.5–0.6 g (wet), 0.1–0.15 g (dry).
- Retina: 0.25–0.3 g (wet), 0.05–0.09 g (dry).
- Sclera: 0.9–1.1 g (wet), 0.2–0.3 g (dry).
- Vitreous Body: 4–5 g.

Temperature

- Aqueous Humor: 36.0°–37.0 °C (96.8–98.6 °F).
- Choroid: 36.0°–37.0 °C (96.8–98.6 °F).
- Cornea: 32.0°–34.0 °C (89.6–93.2 F).
- Lens: 36.0°–37.0 °C (96.8–98.6 °F).
- Retina: 36.5°–37.0 °C (97.7–98.6 °F).
- Sclera: 35.0°–37.0 °C (95–98.6 °F).
- Vitreous: 36.0°–37.0 °C (96.8–98.6 °F).

References

1. American Academy of Ophthalmology. What is considered normal eye pressure range? [Internet]. San Francisco: American Academy of Ophthalmology; 2025 [cited 2025 Aug 20]. Available from: https://glaucoma.org/articles/what-is-considered-normal-eye-pressureGlaucoma Research Foundation
2. Feng MT, Lim L, Tan GS, et al. Anterior chamber depth in normal subjects by rotating Scheimpflug imaging. Br J Ophthalmol. 2011;95(3):382–5. https://doi.org/10.1136/bjo.2009.176063. PMID: 20584896; PMCID: PMC3729361.PMC
3. Camburu G, Sampaio E, Lima J, et al. The measurement of central corneal thickness. J Glaucoma. 2023;32(5):e283–9. https://doi.org/10.1097/IJG.0000000000002063. PMID: 36893311; PMCID: PMC10385715
4. Bhardwaj V, Saha S, Saha K, et al. Axial length, anterior chamber depth—a study in different age groups. Indian J Ophthalmol. 2013;61(11):644–8. https://doi.org/10.4103/0301-4738.121297. PMID: 24212315; PMCID: PMC3843406.PMC
5. Chan A, Lee G, Lee P, et al. Normal macular thickness measurements in healthy eyes. JAMA Ophthalmol. 2006;124(3):319–24. https://doi.org/10.1001/archopht.124.3.319. PMID: 16505107. JAMA Network+1
6. Kim JS, Lee JH, Lee JH, et al. Retinal nerve fiber layer thickness measurement using spectral-domain optical coherence tomography. J Glaucoma. 2010;19(7):453–9. https://doi.org/10.1097/IJG.0b013e3181e3b6d0. PMID: 20531145; PMCID: PMC2868471
7. Caltrider D. Evaluating visual acuity. In: StatPearls [Internet]. Treasure Island (FL): StatPearls Publishing; 2024 [cited 2025 Aug 20]. Available from: https://www.ncbi.nlm.nih.gov/books/NBK564307/NCBI
8. Lim CS, Chew PT, Tan DT. A simple clinical method to measure the optic disc size in glaucoma. Ophthalmology. 1996;103(6):1012–6. https://doi.org/10.1016/S0161-6420(96)30622-2. PMID: 8795768. PubMed
9. American Academy of Ophthalmology. Cup-to-disc ratio. [Internet]. San Francisco: American Academy of Ophthalmology; 2025 [cited 2025 Aug 20]. Available from: https://www.aao.org/education/image/cup-disc-ratio. American Academy of Ophthalmology.
10. American Academy of Ophthalmology. Eye pressure testing. [Internet]. San Francisco: American Academy of Ophthalmology; 2025 [cited 2025 Aug 20]. Available from: https://www.aao.org/eye-health/tips-prevention/eye-pressure-testing. American Academy of Ophthalmology.

M. P. Kelly, *Normal Values in Vision Science*,
https://doi.org/10.1007/978-3-032-18207-4

11. Jones D. Measure axial length to guide myopia management. [Internet]. Review of Myopia Management; 2023 [cited 2025 Aug 20]. Available from: https://reviewofmm.com/shouldnt-we-treat-axial-length-as-essential-in-treating-myopia/Review of Myopia Management+1
12. Dueker DK, Wilson RS, Klyce SD. Corneal thickness measurement in the management of glaucoma. Ophthalmology. 2007;114(2):221–9. https://doi.org/10.1016/j.ophtha.2006.11.008. PMID: 17270583. AAO Journal
13. Almidani L, Kalloniatis M. Biological and methodological variability in retinal nerve fiber layer thickness measurements. Ophthalmol Ther. 2024;13(1):1–13. https://doi.org/10.1007/s40123-024-00456-2. PMID: 36698372. ScienceDirect
14. Lee W, Lee J, Lee J, et al. Estimation of best corrected visual acuity based on deep learning. Sci Rep. 2022;12(1):1–9. https://doi.org/10.1038/s41598-022-22586-2. PMID: 36415874; PMCID: PMC9708284. Nature

Index

M. P. Kelly, *Normal Values in Vision Science*,
https://doi.org/10.1007/978-3-032-18207-4

MIX
Papier aus verantwortungsvollen Quellen
Paper from responsible sources
FSC® C105338

If you have any concerns about our products,
you can contact us on
ProductSafety@springernature.com

In case Publisher is established outside the EU,
the EU authorized representative is:
Springer Nature Customer Service Center GmbH
Europaplatz 3, 69115 Heidelberg, Germany

Printed by Libri Plureos GmbH
in Hamburg, Germany